# COVID Supplements

## © Copyright: Steven Magee 2023

### Edition 1

Cover Picture:   Steven Magee using his continuous positive airway pressure (CPAP) life support machine after being diagnosed with sleep apnea that causes low oxygen during sleep.  He has been diagnosed with 'Small Airways Disease' of the lungs, a common diagnosis in  'Long COVID' patients.  The rear cover shows him researching at the Oregon State Hospital Museum of Mental Health:

https://oshmuseum.org/

# Contents

# Introduction

I developed a flu-like sickness that was followed by years of long COVID symptoms. My mental and physical health seriously degraded after the flu-like sickness and I was largely a medical mystery to the doctors that were treating me. The prescription medications and medical devices would make me sicker, not better.

Using nutritional supplements and lifestyle changes I started to see beneficial health improvements and my health recovered sufficiently to resume a normal life again. I am sharing the fruits of my discoveries with you, so you can work with your doctor on improving your own health. I got smart and my smart techniques are in this book! At the time of writing, the COVID-19 pandemic was in its fourth year and long COVID was prevalent in the population. The nutritional supplements discussed in this book are being linked to improved health outcomes in both conditions.

Scientific research papers that discuss the nutritional supplements I used to improve my health are presented. My supplementation protocols for my long COVID symptoms were developed from medical research that was freely available on the internet. Altitude tests to cause hypoxia throughout the body were performed on the island of Hawaii from 2021 to 2023 to confirm the supplements prevented altitude sickness from the lower atmospheric oxygen levels.

The three supplement protocols detailed in this book were developed during the COVID-19 pandemic. The long COVID symptoms I was displaying significantly subsided by using the three supplement protocols. I have much better mental and physical health today. I look better too!

This book contains the very latest research on health and the human environment. It should be viewed as the current ideas and the contents are subject to review by the medical community. The author and publisher accept no liability whatsoever for any of the contents and the book is published in the spirit of unrestricted access to the latest ideas and medical theories in a changing world. These are experimental health techniques and the long term side effects are unknown.

You should always consult with a licensed and certified medical professional on any aspects of health, sickness or disease.

*"Smart people realize the smartest person that can fix their health issues is themselves!"*

**Steven Magee**

## Nutrition

**Nutritional status of patients with COVID-19**...The relationship between immunity and nutrition is well known...a deficiency of vitamin D or selenium may decrease the immune defenses against COVID-19 and cause progression to severe disease.

https://www.ncbi.nlm.nih.gov/pmc/articles/PMC7418699/

**Long-term effects of malnutrition on severity of COVID-19**...The COVID-19 pandemic is a public health crisis that has the potential to exacerbate worldwide malnutrition...imply higher odds for severe COVID-19 for children between 6 and 17 years with history of malnutrition. Even higher odds of severe COVID-19 exist for adults (with history of malnutrition) between 18 and 79 years. These results indicate that the long-term effect of malnutrition predisposes patients to severe COVID-19 in an age-dependent way.

https://www.ncbi.nlm.nih.gov/pmc/articles/PMC8298504/

**The Role of Nutrition in COVID-19 Susceptibility and Severity of Disease: A Systematic Review**...Many nutrients have powerful immunomodulatory actions with the potential to alter susceptibility to coronavirus disease 2019 (COVID-19) infection, progression to symptoms, likelihood of severe disease, and survival...Given the known impacts of all forms of malnutrition on the immune system, public health strategies to reduce micronutrient deficiencies and undernutrition remain of critical importance. Furthermore, there is strong evidence that prevention of obesity and type 2 diabetes will reduce the risk of serious COVID-19 outcomes.

https://www.ncbi.nlm.nih.gov/pmc/articles/PMC8194602/

### COVID-19: Role of Nutrition and Supplementation

**Supplementation**...current research indicates that supplementation with multiple micronutrients could be considered important both in the prevention and in the management of the COVID-19 infection. Particular attention should be paid to the substances that play an important role in the regulation of the immune response, considering the possibility of reducing the risk of infection, and, at the same time, improving the health status of COVID-19 patients. The micronutrients with the strongest evidence for immune support are vitamins C, D, and zinc. To date, evidence has been published about the pivotal role of vitamin D: Its deficiency has been associated with increased susceptibility to respiratory infections. Considering that the main pathway of the SARS-CoV-2 infection is at the lung level, it is reasonable that the use of vitamin D supplements could improve the health status of COVID-19 patients, reducing the risk of infection for healthy individuals, helping COVID-19 survivors in the recovery of their lifestyle...the role of probiotics should be better studied in order to reduce the adverse effects at gastrointestinal levels of the COVID-19 infection...it is well described that the worst outcomes occur in subjects with one or more comorbidities. Furthermore, each comorbidity is strictly related to metabolic diseases: For example, the overweight or obese subject has a high risk of developing the severe form of SARS-CoV-2 infection. For these reasons, it is important to take into account the influence of lifestyle habits, such as unhealthy diets, on COVID-19 susceptibility and recovery. In addition, the large number of subjects who recover from COVID-19 could lead to a spike in chronic medical diseases. These conditions could be further exacerbated by a poor diet regimen. Therefore, in consideration of the data discussed in this review, it should be recommended that subjects should avoid eating foods containing high amounts of saturated fat and sugar; contrariwise, it is desirable that they consume high amounts of fiber, whole grains, unsaturated fats, and antioxidants to enhance immune function.

https://www.ncbi.nlm.nih.gov/pmc/articles/PMC8002713/

**The Role of Nutrients in Prevention, Treatment and Post-Coronavirus Disease-2019 (COVID-19)**...the safe intake of micro- and/or macro-nutrients can be useful either for preventing infection and supporting the immune response during COVID-19, as well as in the post-acute phase, i.e., "long COVID", that is sometimes characterized by the onset of various long lasting and disabling symptoms. The aim of this review is to focus on the role of nutrient intake during all the different phases of the disease, including prevention, the acute phase, and finally long COVID… In this review we have discussed a number of studies showing that nutrition may play an important role in influencing both the susceptibility and the clinical course of COVID-19 and long COVID, as is already known for other viral diseases. We have shown that nutritional status plays a pivotal role in the function of the immune system, supporting both innate and adaptive immunity, influencing the proliferation and activity of immune cells. Furthermore, we highlighted that nutrients play a role in reducing inflammation. They inhibit leukocyte chemotaxis, inflammatory cytokine production, and T lymphocyte reactivity. Moreover, they give rise to resolvins and protectins, which participate in the resolution of inflammation by normalizing excessive immune reactions. In addition, they are essential for keeping intact and functioning tissue barriers. Finally, some of them seem to influence viral replication and they have even been shown to have a neuroprotective effect in long COVID, by decreasing cognitive decline.

https://www.ncbi.nlm.nih.gov/pmc/articles/PMC8912782/


**Functional food: complementary to fight against COVID-19**...Numerous functional foods can help the body fight COVID-19 through several mechanisms such as the reduced release of pro-inflammatory cytokines, reduced expression of ACE2 receptors in cells, and inhibiting essential enzymes in SARS-CoV-2...A combination of few common foods is sufficient to prevent many diseases and even alleviate symptoms of patients. For example, herbs such as garlic could be easily added to daily meals, improving the utility of such dishes alongside palatability. For example, bioactive compounds in garlic can inhibit the main protease in SARS-CoV-2, reducing the spread of the virus inside the patient's body. Also, the simple and easy addition of beverages such as green tea can be immensely helpful in the prevention of critical life-threatening diseases. Therefore, supplementing expensive drugs and therapy with cost-effective, simple food ingredients may be the best option for many patients, particularly those who cannot afford conventional medical treatments...COVID-19 patients have reported thrombotic complications associated with vitamin D deficiency. Therefore, consuming vitamin D-rich foods such as mushrooms, milk, and egg yolk can help prevent such complications. Minerals such as zinc also decrease COVID-19 infections that reduce autophagy and allow in vitro RdRp activity in SARS-CoV-2. Zinc-rich foods such as eggs modulate the function and abundance of immune cells alongside cytokine production, stimulate autophagy, improve antiviral drugs' efficacy, and inhibit the processing of viral polyproteins.

https://www.ncbi.nlm.nih.gov/pmc/articles/PMC8899455/


**Nutritional status of micronutrients as a possible and modifiable risk factor for COVID-19: a UK perspective**...Recent scientific evidence has indicated that the elderly have increased risk of COVID-19 infections, with over 70s and 80s being hardest hit - especially residents of care homes and in clinical settings, ethnic minorities, people who work indoors and those who are overweight and obese. Other potential risk factors include lack of exposure to sunlight, darker skin pigmentation, co-morbidities, poor diet, certain medications, disadvantaged social and economic status, and lifestyle factors such as smoking and excessive consumption of alcohol. A key question is to understand how and why certain groups of people are more susceptible to COVID-19, whether they have weakened immune systems and what the roles of good nutrition and specific micronutrients are in supporting immune functions. A varied and balanced diet with an abundance of fruits and vegetables and the essential nutrients like vitamin D, vitamin A, B vitamins (folate, vitamin B6 and vitamin

B12), vitamin C and the minerals, Fe, Cu, Se and Zn are all known to contribute to the normal functions of the immune system. Avoidance of deficiencies and identification of suboptimal intakes of these micronutrients in targeted groups of patients and in distinct and highly sensitive populations could help to strengthen the resilience of people to the COVID-19 pandemic.

https://pubmed.ncbi.nlm.nih.gov/32815493/

*"I uncovered extensive malnutrition issues when I was trying to recover from my Long COVID symptoms."*

**Steven Magee**

## <u>Supplements</u>

**Vitamins, supplements and COVID-19: a review of currently available evidence**...Of the vitamins and supplements that were studied, vitamin D presented the most promising data demonstrating significant decreases in oxygen requirements, need for ICU treatment, SARS-CoV-2 RNA test positivity, and mortality. All of these benefits were exhibited in hospitalized patients. Other vitamins and supplements that were evaluated in studies did not demonstrate any statistically significant benefits. Common shortcomings of the articles included generally small sample sizes, varying sites of study (which could determine the virus variant), a lack of standard of care as background therapy, and utilization of doses that were higher than standard.

https://www.ncbi.nlm.nih.gov/pmc/articles/PMC8496749/

**Dietary Supplements in the Time of COVID-19**...Your immune system needs certain vitamins and minerals to work properly. These include vitamin C, vitamin D, and zinc. Herbal supplements, probiotics, and other dietary supplement ingredients might also affect immunity and inflammation.

https://ods.od.nih.gov/factsheets/
DietarySupplementsInTheTimeOfCOVID19-Consumer/

**Dietary Supplements and COVID-19**...Research suggests that certain dietary supplement ingredients might improve immune response and reduce symptoms of some respiratory illnesses, like the common cold and flu. Popular supplement ingredients that are thought to support immune health include vitamin C, vitamin D, zinc, elderberry, echinacea, and probiotics.

https://covid19.nih.gov/news-and-stories/dietary-supplements-and-covid-19

**Immune-boosting role of vitamins D, C, E, zinc, selenium and omega-3 fatty acids: Could they help against COVID-19?**...Undoubtedly, nutrition is a key determinant of maintaining good health. Key dietary components such as vitamins C, D, E, zinc, selenium and the omega 3 fatty acids have well-established immunomodulatory effects, with benefits in infectious disease. Some of these nutrients have also been shown to have a potential role in the management of COVID-19. In this paper, evidence surrounding the role of these dietary components in immunity as well as their specific effect in COVID-19 patients are discussed. In addition, how supplementation of these nutrients may be used as therapeutic modalities potentially to decrease the morbidity and mortality rates of patients with COVID-19 is discussed.

https://pubmed.ncbi.nlm.nih.gov/33308613/

**Evaluation of the relationship between serum levels of zinc, vitamin B12, vitamin D, and clinical outcomes in patients with COVID-19**...it seems that serum levels of 25(OH)D, vitamin B12, and especially zinc at the time of admission can affect clinical outcomes in COVID-19 patients.

https://pubmed.ncbi.nlm.nih.gov/34406674/

**Cohort study to evaluate the effect of vitamin D, magnesium, and vitamin B12 in combination on progression to severe outcomes in older patients with coronavirus (COVID-19)**...A vitamin D / magnesium / vitamin B12 combination in older COVID-19 patients was associated with a significant reduction in the proportion of patients with clinical deterioration requiring oxygen support, intensive care support, or both. This study supports further larger randomized controlled trials to ascertain the full benefit of this combination in ameliorating the severity of COVID-19.

https://www.ncbi.nlm.nih.gov/pmc/articles/PMC7832811/

*"Boosting up the nutritional status of the body during a pandemic is common sense."*

**Steven Magee**

## Multivitamins

**Role of vitamins and minerals as immunity boosters in COVID-19**...the role of vitamins and minerals in the treatment of COVID-19. A deficiency of these vitamins and minerals in the plasma concentration may lead to a reduction in the good performance of the immune system, which is one of the constituents that lead to a poor immune state. This is a narrative review concerning the features of the COVID-19 and data related to the usage of vitamins and minerals as preventive measures to decrease the morbidity and mortality rate in patients with COVID-19...The possible therapeutic benefits of vitamins A, B, C, D, E, and K via immunomodulation in COVID-19 patients have been evaluated and analyzed based on available evidence. Trace elements such as zinc, selenium, manganese, and copper, are essential micronutrients. Antiviral and antioxidant properties are involved in multiple immunomodulatory pathways and improve the body's defence system by different mechanisms. Supplementation of vitamins and micronutrients may have a positive impact on the recovery of COVID-19 infection. However, there is a lack of preclinical and clinical studies associated with vitamins and micronutrients in the management of COVID-19. To explore the possible beneficial role of vitamins and micronutrients in COVID-19 patients, various clinical studies are being carried out. By reviewing various studies, it can be concluded that adequate supplementation of vitamins and micronutrients should be considered to improve SARS- CoV infection outcomes. The current situation has resulted in several highly effective vaccines, and work is being conducted for targeted drug therapy; these are very expensive and complicated processes with a narrow spectrum targeted activity. In contrast, vitamin and micronutrient supplementation is a relatively cost-efficient and easy approach when supported by robust clinical studies, and has possible broad-spectrum activity and potentially long-term health benefits. While considering the health benefit and risk ratio, vitamin and micronutrients are probably justifiable with negligible risks. This is in contrast with the risk associated with novel drugs and some vaccines. Therefore, nutrient supplementations seem to be a promising approach towards SARS-CoV infection.

https://www.ncbi.nlm.nih.gov/pmc/articles/PMC8190991/

**Could Vitamins Help in the Fight Against COVID-19?**...There are limited proven therapeutic options for the prevention and treatment of COVID-19. The role of vitamin and mineral supplementation or "immunonutrition" has previously been explored in a number of clinical trials in intensive care settings, and there are several hypotheses to support their routine use. The aim of this narrative review was to investigate whether vitamin supplementation is beneficial in COVID-19. A systematic search strategy with a narrative literature summary was designed, using the Medline, EMBASE, Cochrane Trials Register, WHO International Clinical Trial Registry, and Nexis media databases. The immune-mediating, antioxidant and antimicrobial roles of vitamins A to E were explored and their potential role in the fight against COVID-19 was evaluated. The major topics extracted for narrative synthesis were physiological and immunological roles of each vitamin, their role in respiratory infections, acute respiratory distress syndrome (ARDS), and COVID-19. Vitamins A to E highlighted potentially beneficial roles in the fight against COVID-19 via antioxidant effects, immunomodulation, enhancing natural barriers, and local paracrine signaling. Level 1 and 2 evidence supports the use of thiamine, vitamin C, and vitamin D in COVID-like respiratory diseases, ARDS, and sepsis. Although there are currently no published clinical trials due to the novelty of SARS-CoV-2 infection, there is pathophysiologic rationale for exploring the use of vitamins in this global pandemic, supported by early anecdotal reports from international groups.

https://pubmed.ncbi.nlm.nih.gov/32842513/

**The impact of vitamin and mineral supplements usage prior to COVID-19 infection on disease severity and hospitalization**...Nutritional status is suggested to be related to the severity of COVID-19 infection...Among the investigated nutrients, the use of vitamin D prior to COVID-19 infection was associated with reduced disease severity and hospitalization.

https://pubmed.ncbi.nlm.nih.gov/35238285/

**Common drugs, vitamins, nutritional supplements and COVID-19 mortality**...Nutritional supplements may increase survival. Mortality in an Italian nursing home during the COVID-19 pandemic was shown to be reduced with vitamin D supplementation. A vitamin D/magnesium/vitamin B12 combination in older-aged COVID-19 patients was associated with a significant reduction in the proportion of patients with clinical deterioration requiring oxygen support, intensive care support, or both. Vitamin D may be a critical host factor to prevent COVID-19, although this hypothesis remains controversial. To prevent the cytokine storm, the use of N-acetylcysteine in both the prevention and adjuvant therapy of COVID-19 has been suggested. https://www.ncbi.nlm.nih.gov/pmc/articles/PMC8323622/

*"The multivitamin is the base supplement to build an effective nutritional supplementing protocol from."*

**Steven Magee**

## B Vitamins

**Be well: A potential role for vitamin B in COVID-19**...Micronutrients, vitamin C and vitamin D have gained much attention during the pandemic because of their anti-inflammatory and immune-supporting properties. Low levels of vitamins D and C result in coagulopathy and suppress the immune system, causing lymphocytopenia. Evidence has shown that the mortality rate is higher in COVID-19 patients with low vitamin D concentrations. Further, vitamin C supplementation increases the oxygenation index in COVID-19 infected patients. Similarly, vitamin B deficiency can significantly impair cell and immune system function, and lead to inflammation due to hyperhomocysteinemia. There is a need to highlight the importance of vitamin B because it plays a pivotal role in cell functioning, energy metabolism, and proper immune function. Vitamin B assists in proper activation of both the innate and adaptive immune responses, reduces pro-inflammatory cytokine levels, improves respiratory function, maintains endothelial integrity, prevents hypercoagulability and can reduce the length of stay in hospital. Therefore, vitamin B status should be assessed in COVID-19 patients and vitamin B could be used as a non-pharmaceutical adjunct to current treatments.

https://www.ncbi.nlm.nih.gov/pmc/articles/PMC7428453/

**The association between B vitamins and the risk of COVID-19**...B vitamins are essential micronutrients for the body with antioxidant, anti-inflammatory and immune-regulating properties...A higher intake of vitamin B5 could reduce the odds of COVID-19 by 47 %, and a moderate intake of vitamin B12 had a protective effect on COVID-19.

https://pubmed.ncbi.nlm.nih.gov/36348570/

*"B vitamins are often called 'Energy' vitamins, as they are known to improve energy levels in people."*

**Steven Magee**

# Vitamin B6

**Potential Role of Vitamin B6 in Ameliorating the Severity of COVID-19 and Its Complications**...Vitamin B6 is a water-soluble vitamin found in various foods such as fish, whole grains, and banana. There are six isoforms of B6 vitamers. Among these, pyridoxal 5'-phosphate is the most active form that acts as a coenzyme in various enzymatic reactions. There is growing evidence that vitamin B6 exerts a protective effect against chronic diseases such as cardiovascular diseases (CVD) and diabetes by suppressing inflammation, inflammasomes, oxidative stress, and carbonyl stress. Additionally, vitamin B6 deficiency is associated with lower immune function and higher susceptibility to viral infection. In view of these information, we postulated potential role of vitamin B6 in ameliorating the severity of COVID-19 and its complications...Accumulating evidence suggests that vitamin B6 supplementation may be useful for COVID-19 patients with low vitamin B6 status.

https://www.ncbi.nlm.nih.gov/pmc/articles/PMC7658555/

**Modeling studies on the role of vitamins B1 (thiamin), B3 (nicotinamide), B6 (pyridoxamine), and caffeine as potential leads for the drug design against COVID-19**...Our results pointed to vitamins B1 and B6 in the neutral form as potential binders to the HssACE2 RDB binding pocket that might be able to impair the SARS-CoV-2 mechanism of cell invasion, qualifying as potential leads for experimental investigation against COVID-19.

https://www.ncbi.nlm.nih.gov/pmc/articles/PMC9640828/

*“Vitamin B6 may boost the immune system.”*
**Steven Magee**

## Biotin (B7)

**Could Vitamins Help in the Fight Against COVID-19?**...vitamin B7 (biotin) is also recognized as an immunoregulatory vitamin through its effects on proinflammatory cytokine expression.

https://www.ncbi.nlm.nih.gov/pmc/articles/PMC7551685/

**Importance of Dietary Changes During the Coronavirus Pandemic: How to Upgrade Your Immune Response**...Vitamin B7 has a crucial role in nutrition and an important effect in immunometabolism. In fact, by being an essential cofactor for acetyl-CoA carboxylase and fatty acid synthase, this vitamin is used by the body to metabolize carbohydrates, fats, and amino acids (229). The AI of vitamin B7 is 12–30 µg/day for adults (150). Vitamin B7 deficiency induces Th1- and Th17-mediated pro-inflammatory responses in human CD4+ T lymphocytes (230). In the same context, a diet rich in vitamin B7 has anti-inflammatory effects and inhibits the activation of the transcription of NF-$\varkappa$B and thus inhibits the secretion of pro-inflammatory cytokines such as TNF-$\alpha$, IL-1, IL-6, and IL-8.

https://www.ncbi.nlm.nih.gov/pmc/articles/PMC7481450/

**The snapshot of metabolic health in evaluating micronutrient status, the risk of infection and clinical outcome of COVID-19**...adequate energy production for immune cell activities, gut microbiota composition, fatty acid oxidation, reactive oxygen species (ROS) generation, T cell differentiation and regulation of inflammatory signaling, all comprise key components of B-vitamin mediated monitoring. The sufficiency of beneficial gut microflora can be indirectly evaluated through the levels of vitamin B7 (biotin). This vitamin is endogenously produced by probiotic gastrointestinal bacteria and is required as a coenzyme to promote fatty acid biosynthesis, gluconeogenesis and amino acid metabolism. Biotin-dependent 3-methylcrotonyl-CoA carboxylase promotes leucine catabolism, and decreased enzymatic capacity is associated with the accumulation of 3-methyl crotonic acid and 3-hydroxyisovaleric acid in the biological fluids.

https://www.ncbi.nlm.nih.gov/pmc/articles/PMC8234252/


**Beneficial Effects of Vitamins, Minerals, and Bioactive Peptides on Strengthening the Immune System Against COVID-19 and the Role of Cow's Milk in the Supply of These Nutrients**...Vitamin B7 (biotin) also affects the expression of proinflammatory cytokines and is considered a vitamin that regulates the immune system.

https://www.ncbi.nlm.nih.gov/pmc/articles/PMC8627168/


*"Vitamin B7 is produced by probiotic gastrointestinal bacteria."*

**Steven Magee**

## Folate (B9)

**Folate Levels in Patients Hospitalized with Coronavirus Disease 2019**...Folic acid (FA), also known as folate, is an essential vitamin vital for human homeostasis, participating in many biochemical pathways, and its deficiency has been associated with viral infection vulnerability...Data from in silico studies and molecular docking support that FA inhibits SARS-CoV-2 entry into the host and viral replication, binding at essential residues. Accordingly, in patients' studies, a protective role of FA supplementation against SARS-CoV-2 infection is indicated.

https://www.ncbi.nlm.nih.gov/pmc/articles/PMC10052526/

**Role of Folate, Cobalamin, and Probiotics in COVID-19 Disease Management [Letter]**...the use of vitamins B9, B12 probiotics, and magnesium, which have also exhibited a positive impact on the prognosis of the infection...Multiple studies have shown that folic acid inhibits the binding of the SARS-CoV-2 spike proteins, which blocks the entry of the virus into the cell. One study suggested that vitamin B9 acted as an inhibitor of the furin enzyme, and thus prevented the virus from entering the cell, and another preprint reported that the derivatives of Folic acid, especially 5-methyl tetrahydrofolic acid and tetrahydrofolic acid, have a strong binding affinity against the SARS-CoV-2...It is evident from the aforementioned studies that there is a significant role of vitamins B9, B12, magnesium, and probiotics in managing the Covid-19 disease.

https://www.ncbi.nlm.nih.gov/pmc/articles/PMC8403566/

**Nutrition in the Actual COVID-19 Pandemic. A Narrative Review**...the data shown indicate that, while the hospitalized patient is not usually deficient in vitamins B1 and B12 or zinc, the vast majority can reveal at least one nutrient deficiency. Specifically, 42% of patients hospitalized for COVID-19 have presented selenium deficiency, 6% of vitamin B6, and 4% of folate...the following nutrients and nutraceuticals have been found to offer a somewhat brain-protective effect. Lipids as Omega-3 fatty acid (Eicosapentaenoic, Docosahexaenoic, Linoleic α-lipoic acids), vitamins (C, B9, D3, and E), Plant polyphenols (Flavone as Apigenin and Luteolin; Flavonol as Tangeretin, Chrysin, Quercetin; Isoflavone as Naringenin, Naringin, Hesperetin, Rutin; Antocyanidines; Phenolic Acids; Stilbene; Trace elements as Theophylline, Capsaicin, Piperine, and Zin; Endogenous antioxidants as Selenium, Glutathione, Melatonin, Creatin, and N-acetyl-cysteine).

https://www.ncbi.nlm.nih.gov/pmc/articles/PMC8228835/

**Folic acid and methotrexate use and their association with COVID-19 diagnosis and mortality: a case control analysis from the UK Biobank**...We report an association of increased risk for COVID-19 diagnosis and COVID-19-related death in people prescribed folic acid supplementation. Our results also suggest that methotrexate might attenuate these associations.

https://www.ncbi.nlm.nih.gov/pmc/articles/PMC9412040/

*"Folic acid deficiency is associated with viral infection vulnerability."*

**Steven Magee**

## Vitamin B12

**The role of vitamin B12 in viral infections: a comprehensive review of its relationship with the muscle–gut–brain axis and implications for SARS-CoV-2 infection**...The evaluation of parameters that determine the deficiency or subclinical levels of vitamin B12 deficiency can be an ally in treating patients affected by COVID-19 or in persistent symptoms of the disease, given the important functions of this vitamin in the skeletal muscle–gut–brain axis.  Vitamin B12 plays an important role in viral infections. The consumption of a healthy diet containing vitamin B12 sources, and especially supplementation with methylcobalamin and cyanocobalamin, are promising alternatives as adjuvants in the treatment of COVID-19, especially in patients with B12 deficiency or deficiency risk.

https://www.ncbi.nlm.nih.gov/pmc/articles/PMC8689946/

**Unravelling Vitamin B12 as a potential inhibitor against SARS-CoV-2: A computational approach**...Vitamins are necessary nutrients for cell growth, function, and development. Furthermore, they play an important role in pathogen defence via cell-mediated responses and boost immunity. Using a computational approach, we intend to identify the probable inhibitory effect of all vitamins on the drug targets of COVID-19. The computational analysis demonstrated that vitamin B12 resulted in depicting suitable significant binding with furin, RNA dependent RNA polymerase (RdRp), Main proteases (Mpro), ORF3a and ORF7a and Vitamin D3 with spike protein and vitamin B9 with non structural protein 3 (NSP3). A detailed examination of vitamins suggests that vitamin B12 may be the component that reduces virulence by blocking furin which is responsible for entry of virus in the host cell. Details from the Molecular Dynamics (MD) simulation study aided in determining vitamin B12 as a possible furin inhibitor.

https://www.ncbi.nlm.nih.gov/pmc/articles/PMC9020503/

**Determination of B Vitamins by Double-Vortex-Ultrasonic Assisted Dispersive Liquid-Liquid Microextraction and Evaluation of their Possible Roles in Susceptibility to COVID-19 Infection: Hybrid Box-Behnken Design and Genetic Algorithm...**The results suggest that vitamin B12 deficiency may decrease the immune system defenses against COVID-19 patients without an underlying disease and cause the disease to become severe.

https://pubmed.ncbi.nlm.nih.gov/34718458/

**Vitamin B12 attenuates leukocyte inflammatory signature in COVID-19 via methyl-dependent changes in epigenetic markings...**COVID-19 induces chromatin remodeling in host immune cells, and it had previously been shown that vitamin B12 downregulates some inflammatory genes via methyl-dependent epigenetic mechanisms. In this work, whole blood cultures from moderate or severe COVID-19 patients were used to assess the potential of B12 as adjuvant drug. The vitamin normalized the expression of a panel of inflammatory genes still dysregulated in the leukocytes despite glucocorticoid therapy during hospitalization. B12 also increased the flux of the sulfur amino acid pathway, that regulates the bioavailability of methyl. Accordingly, B12-induced downregulation of CCL3 strongly and negatively correlated with the hypermethylation of CpGs in its regulatory regions. Transcriptome analysis revealed that B12 attenuates the effects of COVID-19 on most inflammation-related pathways affected by the disease. As far as we are aware, this is the first study to demonstrate that pharmacological modulation of epigenetic markings in leukocytes favorably regulates central components of COVID-19 physiopathology.

https://pubmed.ncbi.nlm.nih.gov/36993968/

**Excessive vitamin B12 and poor outcome in COVID-19 pneumonia**...2% of patients admitted to an Intensive Care Unit (ICU) were Vitamin B12 deficient.  Low plasma vitamin B12 (B12) and folate levels may also be associated with high homocysteine concentration…Patients with poor outcome were significantly older (p = 0.01), had lower P/F ratio (p = 0.01) and higher plasma level of B12 (p = 0.02) compared with those who recovered...A shortage of B vitamins may weaken host immune response...A number of mechanisms can cause high Vitamin B12 levels in our study population: elevated levels of carrier proteins, decreased Vitamin B12 clearance by the liver and decreased uptake by peripheral tissues. However, it is tempting to speculate a correlation with the cytokine storm of the COVID-19 infection to consider a potential role of excessive vitamin B12 on predicting illness outcome.

https://www.ncbi.nlm.nih.gov/pmc/articles/PMC7834259/

*"B12 deficiency may cause the COVID-19 disease to become severe."*

**Steven Magee**

## Vitamin C

**The effect of Vitamin C and Zn supplementation on the immune system and clinical outcomes in COVID-19 patients**...a relation between Vitamin C and Zn deficiency and a reduction in the innate immune response, which can ultimately make patients with COVID-19 more vulnerable to viral infection. As such, adequate intake of Vitamin C and Zn, as an adjunctive therapeutic approach with any necessary pharmacological treatment(s), may be necessary to mitigate the adverse physiological effects of COVID-19…The toxicity of Vitamin C and Zn should also be considered to prevent over-supplementation. Over-supplementation of Vitamin C can lead to oxalate toxicity, while increased Zn intake can reduce immune system function. In summary, Vitamin C and Zn supplementation may be useful in mitigating COVID-19 symptomology.

https://www.ncbi.nlm.nih.gov/pmc/articles/PMC9233349/

**How Nutrition can help to fight against COVID-19 Pandemic**...Nutritional status of individuals has been used as resilience towards destabilization during this COVID-19 pandemic. Optimal nutrition and dietary nutrient intake impact the immune system, therefore the only sustainable way to survive in current context is to strengthen the immune system. There is no evidence found that supplement can cure the immune system except Vit C, which is one of the best way to improve immune system. A proper diet can ensure that the body is in proper state to defeat the virus. However along with the dietary management guidelines the food safety management and good food practices is compulsory. This article explores the importance of nutrition to boost immunity and gives some professional and authentic dietary guidelines about nutrition and food safety to withstand COVID-19.

https://www.ncbi.nlm.nih.gov/pmc/articles/PMC7306972/

**Vitamin C Supplementation for the Treatment of COVID-19: A Systematic Review and Meta-Analysis**...The use of vitamin C reduces hospital mortality. The length of stay in the ICU is longer among patients treated with vitamin C. In terms of patient safety, vitamin C has an acceptable profile. Low doses of vitamin C are effective and safe.

https://www.ncbi.nlm.nih.gov/pmc/articles/PMC9570769/

**The protective role of vitamin C in the management of COVID-19: A Review**...Vitamin C is a robust antioxidant that boosts the immune system of the human body. It helps in normal neutrophil function, scavenging of oxidative species, regeneration of vitamin E, modulation of signaling pathways, activation of pro-inflammatory transcription factors, activation of the signaling cascade, regulation of inflammatory mediators, and phagocytosis and increases neutrophil motility to the site of infection. All of these immunological functions are required for the prevention of COVID-19 infection...Considering the role of vitamin C, it would be imperative to administrate vitamin C for the management of severe COVID-19.

https://www.ncbi.nlm.nih.gov/pmc/articles/PMC8665316/

**Vitamin C and COVID-19**...In numerous animal studies, vitamin C has prevented and alleviated viral and bacterial infections. In a few dozen placebo-controlled trials with humans, vitamin C has shortened infections caused by respiratory viruses, which indicates that the vitamin can also influence viral infections in humans. In critically ill patients, plasma vitamin C levels are commonly very low. Gram doses of vitamin C are needed to increase the plasma vitamin C levels of critically ill patients to the levels of ordinary healthy people. A meta-analysis of 12 trials with 1,766 patients calculated that vitamin C reduced the length of ICU stay on average by 8%. Another meta-analysis found that vitamin C shortened the duration of mechanical ventilation in ICU patients. Two randomized placebo-controlled trials found statistically significant reduction in the mortality of sepsis patients. The effects of vitamin C on acute respiratory distress syndrome (ARDS) frequently complicating COVID-19 pneumonia should be considered. Vitamin C is a safe and inexpensive essential nutrient.

https://pubmed.ncbi.nlm.nih.gov/33537320/

**Unwinding the potentials of vitamin C in COVID-19 and other diseases: An updated review**...The discovery of vitamin C (ascorbic acid) is related to the ancient history of persistent research on the origins of the haemorrhagic disease scurvy. Vitamin C is an important nutrient that aids in a variety of biological and physiological processes. Scientists have been researching the function of vitamin C in the prevention and ailment of sepsis and pneumonia for decades. This has created a potential platform for applying these results to individuals suffering from severe coronavirus infection (COVID-19). Vitamin C's ability to activate and enhance the immune system makes it a promising treatment in the present COVID-19 pandemic. Vitamin C also aids in the activation of vitamin B, the production of certain neurotransmitters, and the transformation of cholesterol into bile acids. Hence, vitamin C is used for the treatment of many diseases...There is a potential role of vitamin C in various diseases including neurodegenerative disorders, COVID-19 and other diseases.

https://www.ncbi.nlm.nih.gov/pmc/articles/PMC9713540/

*"Vitamin C is one of the foundations of human health."*

**Steven Magee**

# Vitamin D

**Effects of Vitamin D Supplementation on COVID-19 Related Outcomes: A Systematic Review and Meta-Analysis**...Vitamin D supplementation was significantly associated with a reduced risk of ICU admission (RR = 0.35, 95% CI: 0.20, 0.62) and mortality (RR = 0.46, 95% CI: 0.30, 0.70). Vitamin D supplementation had no significant impact on the risk of COVID-19 infection, whereas it showed protective effects against mortality and ICU admission in COVID-19 patients.

https://pubmed.ncbi.nlm.nih.gov/35631275/

**Relevance of vitamin D3 in COVID-19 infection**...vitamin D3 as an agent with myriad functions, one of them being immunocompetence and a promising weapon for both innate and adaptive immunity against COVID-19 infection. Some of the manifestations of SARS-CoV-2 virus such as Acute Respiratory Distress Syndrome (ARDS) overlap with the pathophysiological effects that are overcome due to already established role of vitamin D3 e.g., amelioration of cytokine outburst. Additionally, the cardiovascular complications due to COVID-19 infection may also be connected to vitamin D3 levels and the activity of its active forms...vitamin D3 deficiency is related to COVID-19 disease. The role that vitamin D3 plays besides its classical actions in immune cells and non-skeletal target tissues would help in extrapolating its role in the severity of this disease and its clinical outcome. At the time of writing this article clinical trials have already been conducted and many more are under way linking the impact of vitamin D3 supplementation and 25(OH)D3 levels on patients with COVID-19 disease. So, until we may find something conclusive it would not be an exaggeration if we state that maintaining the balanced levels of vitamin D3 is highly recommended considering its diverse benefits in our system.

https://www.ncbi.nlm.nih.gov/pmc/articles/PMC8260490/

**Protective Effect of Vitamin D Supplementation on COVID-19-Related Intensive Care Hospitalization and Mortality: Definitive Evidence from Meta-Analysis and Trial Sequential Analysis**...Various studies have found an association between severe vitamin D deficiency and COVID-19-related outcomes. Vitamin D plays a crucial role in immune function and inflammation. Recent data have suggested a protective role of vitamin D in COVID-19-related health outcomes...a definitive association between the protective role of vitamin D and ICU hospitalization.

https://www.ncbi.nlm.nih.gov/pmc/articles/PMC9864223/

**Evidence Regarding Vitamin D and Risk of COVID-19 and Its Severity**...Vitamin D deficiency co exists in patients with COVID-19. At this time, dark skin color, increased age, the presence of pre-existing illnesses and vitamin D deficiency are features of severe COVID disease. Of these, only vitamin D deficiency is modifiable. Through its interactions with a multitude of cells, vitamin D may have several ways to reduce the risk of acute respiratory tract infections and COVID-19: reducing the survival and replication of viruses, reducing risk of inflammatory cytokine production, increasing angiotensin-converting enzyme 2 concentrations, and maintaining endothelial integrity. Fourteen observational studies offer evidence that serum 25-hydroxyvitamin D concentrations are inversely correlated with the incidence or severity of COVID-19...the evidence seems strong enough that people and physicians can use or recommend vitamin D supplements to prevent or treat COVID-19 in light of their safety and wide therapeutic window.

https://pubmed.ncbi.nlm.nih.gov/33142828/

*"It took several months of high dosing with vitamin D to raise my levels from the low to high end of the medical testing range."*

**Steven Magee**

## Vitamin E

**The effect of supplementation with vitamins A, B, C, D, and E on disease severity and inflammatory responses in patients with COVID-19: a randomized clinical trial**...The intervention group (n=30) received vitamins, and the control group did not receive any vitamin or placebo. The intervention was included 25,000 IU daily of vitamins A, 600,000 IU once during the study of D, 300 IU twice daily of E, 500 mg four times daily of C, and one amp daily of B complex for 7 days...The effect of vitamins on the mortality rate was not statistically significant (p=0.112). The prolonged hospitalization rate to more than 7 days was significantly lower in the intervention group than the control group (p=0.001)...Supplementation with vitamins A, B, C, D, and E could improve the inflammatory response and decrease the severity of disease in ICU-admitted patients with COVID-19.

https://pubmed.ncbi.nlm.nih.gov/34776002/

**Immune-boosting role of vitamins D, C, E, zinc, selenium and omega-3 fatty acids: Could they help against COVID-19?**...The anti-oxidant Vitamin E, and trace element selenium, are major components of anti-oxidant defense. Epidemiological studies demonstrate that deficiencies in either of these nutrients alters immune responses and viral pathogenicity. It has been noted, that there is a correlation between geographic selenium levels and COVID-19 cure rates in different Chinese provinces. Vitamin E and selenium both act through anti-oxidant pathways to increase the number of T cells, enhance mitogenic lymphocyte responses, increase IL-2 cytokine secretion, enhances NK cell activity, and, decreases the risk of infection. Selenium and vitamin E supplementation has also been shown to increase resistance to respiratory infections. It is worthy to note that mixed tocopherols are more effective than α-tocopherol alone, due to the range of receptors for these nutrients.  Despite these beneficial roles in immunity, there is limited information on the effects of vitamin E or selenium supplementation in humans with COVID-19 infection, though patients are encouraged to have adequate intakes of these antioxidant nutrients...Adequate levels of vitamins C, D and E are crucial during COVID-19 to reduce symptom burden and lessen the duration of respiratory infection.

https://www.ncbi.nlm.nih.gov/pmc/articles/PMC7415215/

*"There is little information available on the role of vitamin E to treat COVID-19."*

**Steven Magee**

## Calcium

**Low serum calcium: a new, important indicator of COVID-19 patients from mild/moderate to severe/critical...** Our finding indicates that calcium balance is a primal hit of COVID-19 and a biomarker of clinical severity at the beginning of symptom onset. Calcium is closely associated with virus-associated multiple organ injuries and the increase in inflammatory cytokines. Our results provide a new, important indicator of COVID-19 patients from mild/moderate to severe/critical: serum calcium.

https://www.ncbi.nlm.nih.gov/pmc/articles/PMC7755121/

**Conflicts over calcium and the treatment of COVID-19...**Several recent studies have provided evidence that use of calcium channel blockers (CCBs), especially amlodipine and nifedipine, can reduce mortality from coronavirus disease 2019 (COVID-19). Moreover, hypocalcemia (a reduced level of serum ionized calcium) has been shown to be strongly positively associated with COVID-19 severity. Both effectiveness of CCBs as antiviral therapy, and positive associations of hypocalcemia with mortality, have been demonstrated for many other viruses as well. We evaluate these findings in the contexts of virus–host evolutionary conflicts over calcium metabolism, and hypocalcemia as either pathology, viral manipulation or host defence against pathogens. Considerable evidence supports the hypothesis that hypocalcemia represents a host defence. Indeed, hypocalcemia may exert antiviral effects in a similar manner as do CCBs, through interference with calcium metabolism in virus-infected cells. Prospective clinical studies that address the efficacy of CCBs and hypocalcemia should provide novel insights into the pathogenicity and treatment of COVID-19 and other viruses.

https://www.ncbi.nlm.nih.gov/pmc/articles/PMC7717197/

**Serum vitamin D, calcium, and zinc levels in patients with COVID-19**...The results showed that serum of Zinc, calcium, and vitamin D levels in COVID-19 patients are lower than in healthy individuals. So, such nutrients are characterized to be widely available, safe, and low-cost measure that helps cope with the increased demand for these nutrients in case of contact with the virus and onset of the immune responses. They also lower the risk of severe progression and prognosis of this viral infection.

https://www.ncbi.nlm.nih.gov/pmc/articles/PMC8053215/

**The effect of low serum calcium level on the severity and mortality of Covid patients: A systematic review and meta-analysis**...Based on the results of meta-analysis in people with lower calcium, mortality and complications are higher, therefore, serum calcium is a prognostic factor in determining the severity of the disease. Consequently, it is suggested that serum calcium levels should be considered in initial assessments.

https://pubmed.ncbi.nlm.nih.gov/34534417/

*"Low calcium is characteristic of COVID-19."*

**Steven Magee**

# Iron

**Anemia and iron metabolism in COVID-19: a systematic review and meta-analysis**...Iron metabolism and anemia may play an important role in multiple organ dysfunction syndrome in Coronavirus disease 2019 (COVID-19)...Hemoglobin levels were lower with older age, higher percentage of subjects with diabetes, hypertension and overall comorbidities, and admitted to intensive care. Ferritin level increased with older age, increasing proportion of hypertensive study participants, and increasing proportion of mortality...A significant difference in mean ferritin levels of 606.37 ng/mL (95% CI 461.86; 750.88) was found between survivors and non-survivors, but not in hemoglobin levels.

https://pubmed.ncbi.nlm.nih.gov/32816244/

**Iron and iron-related proteins in COVID-19**...COVID-19 pathogenesis involves alteration in iron homeostasis… Hemoglobin levels can be low or normal, and compromised hemoglobin function has been proposed. Membrane-bound transferrin receptor may facilitate viral entry, so it acts as a potential target for antiviral therapy. Lactoferrin can provide natural defense by preventing viral entry and/or inhibiting viral replication. Serum iron and ferritin levels can predict COVID-19-related hospitalization, severity, and mortality. Serum hepcidin and ferritin/transferrin ratio can predict COVID-19 severity.

https://www.ncbi.nlm.nih.gov/pmc/articles/PMC9289930/

**Iron metabolism in infections: Focus on COVID-19**...The COVID-19 pandemic has boosted research on multiple aspects of immunology, including nutritional immunity. Iron is emerging as an important player to ensure an adequate immune response, and studies on iron metabolism in COVID-19 have highlighted a number of interesting intersections. While several studies have established the functional implications of the battle for iron between bacteria, certain parasites, and the host, the scenario is less clear in viral infections. Indeed, distinct patterns of hepcidin and iron regulation have been reported to occur during different viral infections. Severe COVID-19 appears to be characterized by high hepcidin and marked functional iron deficiency, the latter being possibly related to impaired response to hypoxia and lymphocyte function...Assuming COVID-19 as a valuable model, further studies are needed to better clarify the role of altered iron metabolism in severe viral infections and hyperinflammatory syndromes, possibly paving the way to new therapeutic approaches.

https://www.ncbi.nlm.nih.gov/pmc/articles/PMC8305218/

**Association between iron metabolism and SARS-COV-2 infection, determined by ferritin, hephaestin and hypoxia-induced factor-1 alpha levels in COVID-19 patients**...Levels of hephaestin and HIF-1α were found to be inversely related levels of ferritin across all participants in the study, and to our knowledge this is the first report of hephaestin and HIF-1α as potential markers of iron status.

https://www.ncbi.nlm.nih.gov/pmc/articles/PMC9812738/

**The Impact of Iron Dyshomeostasis and Anaemia on Long-Term Pulmonary Recovery and Persisting Symptom Burden after COVID-19: A Prospective Observational Cohort Study**...Coronavirus disease 2019 (COVID-19) is frequently associated with iron dyshomeostasis. The latter is related to acute disease severity and COVID-19 convalescence...At 60 days post-COVID-19 follow-up, hyperferritinaemia (35% of patients), iron deficiency (24% of the cohort) and anaemia (9% of the patients) were frequently found. Anaemia of inflammation (AI) was the predominant feature at early post-acute follow-up, whereas the anaemia phenotype shifted towards iron deficiency anaemia (IDA) and combinations of IDA and AI until the 360 days follow-up. The prevalence of anaemia significantly decreased over time, but iron dyshomeostasis remained a frequent finding throughout the study. Neither iron dyshomeostasis nor anaemia were related to persisting structural lung impairment, but both were associated with impaired stress resilience at long-term COVID-19 follow-up. To conclude, iron dyshomeostasis and anaemia are frequent findings after COVID-19 and may contribute to its long-term symptomatic outcome.

https://www.ncbi.nlm.nih.gov/pmc/articles/PMC9228477/

*"Iron dyshomeostasis and anaemia are common after COVID-19 infection."*

**Steven Magee**

## Magnesium

**Higher Intake of Dietary Magnesium Is Inversely Associated With COVID-19 Severity and Symptoms in Hospitalized Patients: A Cross-Sectional Study**...We found that higher intake of dietary magnesium was inversely associated with COVID-19 severity and symptoms.

https://www.ncbi.nlm.nih.gov/pmc/articles/PMC9132593/

**Magnesium-to-Calcium Ratio and Mortality from COVID-19**...Obesity, type 2 diabetes, arterial hypertension, decrease in immune response, cytokine storm, endothelial dysfunction, and arrhythmias, which are frequent in COVID-19 patients, are associated with hypomagnesemia. Given that cellular influx and efflux of magnesium and calcium involve the same transporters, we aimed to evaluate the association of serum magnesium-to-calcium ratio with mortality from severe COVID-19...our results show that a magnesium-to-calcium ratio ≤0.20 is strongly associated with mortality in patients with severe COVID-19.

https://www.ncbi.nlm.nih.gov/pmc/articles/PMC9101802/

**The relevance of magnesium homeostasis in COVID-19**...existing data seem to corroborate an association between deranged magnesium homeostasis and COVID-19, and call for further and better studies to explore the prophylactic or therapeutic potential of magnesium supplementation...We propose to reconsider the relevance of magnesium, frequently overlooked in clinical practice. Therefore, magnesemia should be monitored and, in case of imbalanced magnesium homeostasis, an appropriate nutritional regimen or supplementation might contribute to protect against SARS-CoV-2 infection, reduce severity of COVID-19 symptoms and facilitate the recovery after the acute phase.

https://www.ncbi.nlm.nih.gov/pmc/articles/PMC8540865/

**Can Maintaining Optimal Magnesium Balance Reduce the Disease Severity of COVID-19 Patients?**...Magnesium is an essential nutrient that has many studied benefits in humans. This brief commentary aims to describe the potential benefits of magnesium on COVID-19 patients and the reported effects of low versus high magnesium levels in SARS−CoV−2 infected individuals. Also, the potential benefits of vitamin D and how magnesium acts as a cofactor to activate vitamin D functions are elaborated. The results of the existing studies point towards evidence that magnesium may have significant benefits in reducing the severity of COVID-19 symptoms. There is also evidence that magnesium-dependent vitamin D activities may have antiviral effects, thus potentially being able to reduce rates of COVID-19 infection, which is a hypothesis that should be further tested…Basic nutrients that optimize physiologic functions in the body, such as magnesium, may be used as a prophylactic measure that can improve patient outcomes in individuals infected by SARS−CoV−2, and potentially even reduce the intensity of the infection by the virus by potentiating vitamin D functions. In the U.S., more than 50% of people are magnesium deficient, and magnesium deficiency is also prevalent in many other countries. The low level of magnesium in the general population may make individuals more vulnerable to viral insults. The high prevalence of magnesium deficiency makes it important to determine how optimal and suboptimal magnesium levels affect COVID-19 patient outcomes.

https://www.ncbi.nlm.nih.gov/pmc/articles/PMC9001958/

**Prognostic Value of Magnesium in COVID-19: Findings from the COMEPA Study**...Magnesium (Mg) plays a key role in infections. However, its role in coronavirus disease 2019 (COVID-19) is still underexplored, particularly in long-term sequelae. The aim of the present study was to examine the prognostic value of serum Mg levels in older people affected by

COVID-19. Patients were divided into those with serum Mg levels ≤1.96 vs. >1.96 mg/dL, according to the Youden index. A total of 260 participants (mean age 65 years, 53.8% males) had valid Mg measurements. Serum Mg had a good accuracy in predicting in-hospital mortality (area under the curve = 0.83; 95% CI: 0.74-0.91). Low serum Mg at admission significantly predicted in-hospital death (HR = 1.29; 95% CI: 1.03-2.68) after adjusting for several confounders. A value of Mg ≤ 1.96 mg/dL was associated with a longer mean length of stay compared to those with a serum Mg > 1.96 (15.2 vs. 12.7 days). Low serum Mg was associated with a higher incidence of long COVID symptomatology (OR = 2.14; 95% CI: 1.30-4.31), particularly post-traumatic stress disorder (OR = 2.00; 95% CI: 1.24-16.40). In conclusion, low serum Mg levels were significant predictors of mortality, length of stay, and onset of long COVID symptoms, indicating that measuring serum Mg in COVID-19 may be helpful in the prediction of complications related to the disease.

https://pubmed.ncbi.nlm.nih.gov/36839188/

*"Higher magnesium levels are associated with better COVID-19 outcomes."*

**Steven Magee**

## Zinc

**Low Levels of Few Micronutrients May Impact COVID-19 Disease Progression: An Observational Study on the First Wave**...Low levels of vitamin A and zinc are associated with a greater need for admission to the ICU and orotracheal intubation. Patients older than 65 years had higher mortality. Randomized clinical trials are needed to examine whether micronutrient supplementation could be beneficial as an adjunctive treatment in COVID-19.

https://www.ncbi.nlm.nih.gov/pmc/articles/PMC8467487/

**Zinc supplementation and COVID-19 mortality: a meta-analysis**...Zinc supplementation can reduce mortality in patients with severe pneumonia...This meta-analysis has suggested that zinc supplementation is associated with a lower mortality rate in COVID-19 patients. Zinc supplementation could be considered as a simple way and cost benefit approach for reduction of mortality in COVID-19 patients.

https://pubmed.ncbi.nlm.nih.gov/35599332/

**Zinc role in Covid-19 disease and prevention**...Zinc (Zn) is a very valuable metal because of its many functions.  It maintains the neurological, immune, reproductive, and skin systems.  Zn involves in enzyme catalysis, protein-protein functions, and protein oligonucleotide maintenance.  The intracellular Zn is connected to metallothionein (MT). This controls the Zn levels through an intracellular process.  Zn modulation of MT mRNA expression is known.  Zn modulates mRNA levels of cytokines. It down-regulates microRNA expression and key enzymes and proteins necessary for microRNA maturation and stability.  Zn concentration in cells is controlled by homeostasis which helps the organism to accumulate diverse dietary Zn. Zn enables the body to make proteins and DNA. It promotes wound healing. It is important in childhood growth and development. It also has antioxidant properties. Zn is also important in cell-mediated immune function. Zn may reduce the duration of cold symptoms, support blood sugar control, improve severe and inflammatory acne, decrease heart disease risk, and slow the progression of macular degeneration. Zn has also been shown to regulate gene transcription in cancer cells. Zn is an anti-inflammatory and detox compound that also helps as detailed later with Covid-19 infection in prophylaxis and treatment. It may thus also improve the efficacy, as well as reduce inflammation and toxic effects of Covid-19 vaccines...Zn is certainly not a 100% effective therapy for Covid-19 infection. However, it has been shown that Zn help with Covid-19 infection. Zn deficiency has been associated with more serious consequences of Covid-19 infection. Zn supplementation is important in the prevention, as well as the treatment in conjunction with antivirals such as Chloroquine or Hydroxychloroquine. Regarding Zn Covid-19 studies,17 reports of 15 studies where it is shown Zn supplementation matters in different phases of Covid-19 infection...Supplementation by vitamins and minerals, in general, may also help to make vaccines more effective. Supplementation with Vitamins B6 and E, Zn, and selenium in elderly people improves their immune system response to challenges.

https://www.ncbi.nlm.nih.gov/pmc/articles/PMC9374320/


**Zinc and COVID-19: Immunity, Susceptibility, Severity and Intervention**...During the coronavirus disease 2019 (COVID-19) pandemic and continuing emergence of viral mutants, there has been a lack of effective treatment methods. Zinc maintains immune function, with direct and indirect antiviral activities. Zinc nutritional status is a critical factor in antiviral immune responses. Importantly, COVID-19 and zinc deficiency overlap in high-risk population. Hence, the potential effect of zinc as a preventive and adjunct therapy for COVID-19 is intriguing. Here, this review summarizes the immune and antiviral function of zinc, the relationship between zinc levels, susceptibility, and severity of COVID-19, and the effect of zinc supplementation on

COVID-19. Existing studies have confirmed that zinc deficiency was associated with COVID-19 susceptibility and severity. Zinc supplementation plays a potentially protective role in enhancing immunity, decreasing susceptibility, shortening illness duration, and reducing the severity of COVID-19. We recommend that zinc levels should be monitored, particularly in COVID-19 patients, and zinc as a preventive and adjunct therapy for COVID-19 should be considered for groups at risk of zinc deficiency to reduce susceptibility and disease severity.

https://pubmed.ncbi.nlm.nih.gov/36094452/

*"Zinc is a potent antiviral."*

**Steven Magee**

# Alpha Lipoic Acid (ALA)

**Mechanics Insights of Alpha-Lipoic Acid against Cardiovascular Diseases during COVID-19 Infection**...Cardiovascular complications are rapidly emerging as a major peril in COVID-19 in addition to respiratory disease. The mechanisms underlying the excessive effect of severe acute respiratory syndrome coronavirus 2 (SARS-CoV-2) infection on patients with cardiovascular comorbidities remain only partly understood. SARS-CoV-2 infection is caused by binding of the viral surface spike (S) protein to the human angiotensin-converting enzyme 2 (ACE2), followed by the activation of the S protein by transmembrane protease serine 2 (TMPRSS2). ACE2 is expressed in the lung (mainly in type II alveolar cells), heart, blood vessels, small intestine, etc., and appears to be the predominant portal to the cellular entry of the virus. Based on current information, most people infected with SARS-CoV-2 virus have a good prognosis, while a few patients reach critical condition, especially the elderly and those with chronic underlying diseases. The "cytokine storm" observed in patients with severe COVID-19 contributes to the destruction of the endothelium, leading to "acute respiratory distress syndrome" (ARDS), multiorgan failure, and death. At the origin of the general proinflammatory state may be the SARS-CoV-2-mediated redox status in endothelial cells via the upregulation of ACE/Ang II/AT1 receptors pathway or the increased mitochondrial reactive oxygen species (mtROS) production. Furthermore, this vicious circle between oxidative stress (OS) and inflammation induces endothelial dysfunction, endothelial senescence, high risk of thrombosis and coagulopathy. The microvascular dysfunction and the formation of microthrombi in a way differentiate the SARS-CoV-2 infection from the other respiratory diseases and bring it closer to cardiovascular diseases like myocardial infarction and stroke. Due the role played by OS in the evolution of viral infection and in the development of COVID-19 complications, the use of antioxidants as adjuvant therapy seems appropriate in this new pathology. Alpha-lipoic acid (ALA) could be a promising candidate that, through its wide tissue distribution and versatile antioxidant properties, interferes with several signaling pathways. Thus, ALA improves endothelial function by restoring the endothelial nitric oxide synthase activity and presents an anti-inflammatory effect dependent or independent of its antioxidant properties. By improving mitochondrial function, it can sustain the tissues' homeostasis in critical situation and by enhancing the reduced glutathione it could indirectly strengthen the immune system. This complex analysis could open a new therapeutic perspective for ALA in COVID-19 infection.

https://www.ncbi.nlm.nih.gov/pmc/articles/PMC8348748/

**The effects of lipoic acid on respiratory diseases**...Respiratory diseases, including lung cancer, pulmonary fibrosis, asthma, and the recently emerging fatal coronavirus disease-19 (COVID-19), are the leading causes of illness and death worldwide. The increasing incidence and mortality rates have attracted much attention to the prevention and treatment of these conditions. Lipoic acid (LA), a naturally occurring organosulfur compound, is not only essential for mitochondrial aerobic metabolism but also shows therapeutic potential via certain pharmacological effects (e.g., antioxidative and anti-inflammatory effects). In recent years, accumulating evidence (animal experiments and in vitro studies) has suggested a role of LA in ameliorating many respiratory diseases (e.g., lung cancer, fibrosis, asthma, acute lung injury and smoking-induced lung injury). Therefore, this review will provide an overview of the present investigational evidence on the therapeutic effect of LA against respiratory diseases in vitro and in vivo.

https://www.ncbi.nlm.nih.gov/pmc/articles/PMC9933494/

**Molecular and Therapeutic Insights of Alpha-Lipoic Acid as a Potential Molecule for Disease Prevention**...Alpha-lipoic acid is an organic, sulfate-based compound produced by plants, humans, and animals. As a potent antioxidant and a natural dithiol compound, it performs a crucial role in mitochondrial bioenergetic reactions. A healthy human body, on the other hand, can synthesize enough α-lipoic acid to scavenge reactive oxygen species and increase endogenous antioxidants; however, the amount of α-lipoic acid inside the body decreases significantly with age, resulting in endothelial dysfunction. Molecular orbital energy and spin density analysis indicate that the sulfhydryl (-SH) group of molecules has the greatest electron donating activity, which would be responsible for the antioxidant potential and free radical scavenging activity. α-Lipoic acid acts as a chelating agent for metal ions, a quenching agent for reactive oxygen species, and a reducing agent for the oxidized form of glutathione and vitamins C and E. α-Lipoic acid enantiomers and its reduced form have antioxidant, cognitive, cardiovascular, detoxifying, anti-aging, dietary supplement, anti-cancer, neuroprotective, antimicrobial, and anti-inflammatory properties. α-Lipoic acid has cytotoxic and antiproliferative effects on several cancers, including polycystic ovarian syndrome. It also has usefulness in the context of female and male infertility. Although α-lipoic acid has numerous clinical applications, the majority of them stem from its antioxidant properties; however, its bioavailability in its pure form is low (approximately 30%). However, nanoformulations have shown promise in this regard. The proton affinity and electron donating activity, as a redox-active agent, would be responsible for the antioxidant potential and free radical scavenging activity of the molecule. This review discusses the most recent clinical data on α-lipoic acid in the prevention, management, and treatment of a variety of diseases, including coronavirus disease 2019.

https://www.ncbi.nlm.nih.gov/pmc/articles/PMC9904877/


**A Combination of α-Lipoic Acid (ALA) and Palmitoylethanolamide (PEA) Blocks Endotoxin-Induced Oxidative Stress and Cytokine Storm: A Possible Intervention for COVID-19**...The global scientific community is striving to understand the pathophysiological mechanisms and develop effective therapeutic strategies for COVID-19. Despite overwhelming data, there is limited knowledge about the molecular mechanisms involved in the prominent cytokine storm syndrome and multiple organ failure and fatality in COVID-19 cases. The aim of this work is to investigate the possible role of of α-lipoic acid (ALA) and palmitoylethanolamide (PEA), in countering the mechanisms in overproduction of reactive oxygen species (ROS), and inflammatory cytokines. An in vitro model of lipopolysaccharide (LPS)-stimulated human epithelial lung cells that mimics the pathogen-associated molecular pattern and reproduces the cell signaling pathways in cytokine storm syndrome has been used. In this model of acute lung injury, the combination effects of ALAPEA, administered before and after LPS injury, were investigated. Our data demonstrated that a combination of 50 μM ALA + 5 μM PEA can reduce ROS and nitric oxide (NO) levels modulating the major cytokines involved on COVID-19 infection when administered either before or after LPS-induced damage. The best outcome was observed when administered after LPS, thus reinforcing the hypothesis that ALA combined with PEA to modulate the key point of cytokine storm syndrome. This work supports for the first time that the combination of ALA with PEA may represent a novel intervention strategy to counteract inflammatory damage related to COVID-19 by restoring the cascade activation of the immune response and acting as a powerful antioxidant.

https://pubmed.ncbi.nlm.nih.gov/34405764/

*"Lipoic Acid is used to treat respiratory diseases."*

**Steven Magee**

## Female Hormones

**Estrogen and COVID-19 symptoms: Associations in women from the COVID Symptom Study**...It has been widely observed that adult men of all ages are at higher risk of developing serious complications from COVID-19 when compared with women. This study aimed to investigate the association of COVID-19 positivity and severity with estrogen exposure in women, in a population based matched cohort study of female users of the COVID Symptom Study application in the UK. Analyses included 152,637 women for menopausal status, 295,689 women for exogenous estrogen intake in the form of the combined oral contraceptive pill (COCP), and 151,193 menopausal women for hormone replacement therapy (HRT). Data were collected using the COVID Symptom Study in May-June 2020. Analyses investigated associations between predicted or tested COVID-19 status and menopausal status, COCP use, and HRT use, adjusting for age, smoking and BMI, with follow-up age sensitivity analysis, and validation in a subset of participants from the TwinsUK cohort. Menopausal women had higher rates of predicted COVID-19 ($P = 0.003$). COCP-users had lower rates of predicted COVID-19 ($P = 8.03E-05$), with reduction in hospital attendance ($P = 0.023$). Menopausal women using HRT or hormonal therapies did not exhibit consistent associations, including increased rates of predicted COVID-19 ($P = 2.22E-05$) for HRT users alone. The findings support a protective effect of estrogen exposure on COVID-19, based on positive association between predicted COVID-19 with menopausal status, and negative association with COCP use. HRT use was positively associated with COVID-19, but the results should be considered with caution due to lack of data on HRT type, route of administration, duration of treatment, and potential unaccounted for confounders and comorbidities.

https://www.ncbi.nlm.nih.gov/pmc/articles/PMC8432854/

**Reflections and recommendations on the COVID-19 pandemic: Should hormone therapy be discontinued?**...At first sight, indications for COVID-19-positive individuals to withdraw from hormone therapy or oral contraceptives may seem a wise recommendation, but it is not based on real data. It takes into consideration only one side of the coin, the procoagulant activity of exogenous oral estrogens. This effect for COVID-19 patients is likely the least important. In these individuals, increased coagulation is consequent to massive endothelial disruption and to the activation of the extrinsic coagulation cascade, with no evidence that an increase in coagulating factors plays any role. By contrast, the advice to withdraw from estrogens misses a consideration of the main effect of estrogens, i.e. their ability to stimulate ACE2 enzyme expression, a critical factor in reducing mortality from COVID-19.

https://www.ncbi.nlm.nih.gov/pmc/articles/PMC7301099/

**Should estrogen be used in the co-treatment of COVID-19 patients? What is the rationale?**...We have read the recommendations from the Spanish Menopause Society regarding the cessation of menopausal hormone therapy (MHT) in order to prevent the execerbation of TE events in COVID-19 patients...we do not recommend cessation of MHT for postmenopausal women with mild or moderate symptoms of COVID-19. Estrogen would prevent the inflammation and the cytokine storm for women with COVID-19. Transdermal application of estrogen may be preferred to oral administration, and transdermal application of estrogen may even be thought of as a co-treatment for COVID-19 with anti-virals and anti-coagulants in postmenopausal women who were not previously users of MHT. However, we do not have sufficient evidence to recommend cessation of MHT in cases of severe COVID-19.

https://www.ncbi.nlm.nih.gov/pmc/articles/PMC7832263/

**The Looming Effects of Estrogen in Covid-19: A Rocky Rollout**...In the face of the Covid-19 pandemic, an intensive number of studies have been performed to understand in a deeper way the mechanisms behind better or worse clinical outcomes. Epidemiologically, men subjects are more prone to severe acute respiratory syndrome-coronavirus type 2 (SARS-CoV-2) infections than women, with a similar scenario being also stated to the previous coronavirus diseases, namely, SARS-CoV in 2003 and Middle East Respiratory Syndrome coronavirus diseases (MERS-CoV) in 2012. In addition, and despite that aging is regarded as an independent risk factor for the severe form of the disease, even so, women protection is evident. In this way, it has been expected that sex hormones are the main determinant factors in gender differences, with the immunomodulatory effects of estrogen in different viral infections, chiefly in Covid-19, attracting more attention as it might explain the case-fatality rate and predisposition of men for Covid-19 severity. Here, we aim to provide a mini-review and an overview on the protective effects of estrogen in Covid-19. Different search strategies were performed including Scopus, Web of Science, Medline, Pubmed, and Google Scholar database to find relative studies. Findings of the present study illustrated that women have a powerful immunomodulating effect against Covid-19 through the effect of estrogen. This study illustrates that estrogens have noteworthy anti-inflammatory and immuno-modulatory effects in Covid-19. Also, estrogen hormone reduces SARS-CoV-2 infectivity through modulation of pro-inflammatory signaling pathways. This study highlighted the potential protective effect of estrogen against Covid-19

https://pubmed.ncbi.nlm.nih.gov/33816542/


**Succinate-Based Dietary Supplement for Menopausal Symptoms: A Pooled Analysis of Two Identical Randomized, Double-Blind, Placebo-Controlled Clinical Trials**...To evaluate the efficacy of a succinate-based dietary supplement (SBDS; Amberen) in symptomatic menopausal women using a larger sample size derived by pooling data from two identical trials...SBDS use resulted in significant improvements in several endpoints including alleviation of 16 of 21 menopausal symptoms (p ≤ 0.05, Greene Scale) and a decrease in anxiety (p < 0.0001,

State-Trait Anxiety Inventory) when compared to placebo. Significant reductions were observed in weight, body mass index, and waist and hip circumferences in the supplement cohort. Evaluation of physiological parameters showed a significant increase in serum estradiol levels compared to baseline ($p < 0.0001$) among users of the SBDS. Levels of follicle stimulating hormone and luteinizing hormone decreased slightly in both groups, without significant differences between the groups. Leptin levels decreased with statistical significance in the SBDS cohort compared to placebo ($p=0.027$). For those with initial leptin concentrations above the reference range, leptin decreased significantly in the SBDS group compared to the baseline ($p < 0.0001$) and to placebo ($p=0.027$)…The pooled analysis reaffirms the outcomes from the individual trials. A nonhormonal, succinate-based dietary supplement is shown to relieve menopausal symptoms when compared to a placebo regimen in a randomized, double-blinded clinical trial.

https://www.ncbi.nlm.nih.gov/pmc/articles/PMC6875258/

*"Estrogen appears to be protective against the damaging effects of COVID-19."*

**Steven Magee**

## Male Hormones

**Testosterone in males with COVID-19: A 7-month cohort study**...Circulating testosterone levels have been found to be reduced in men with severe acute respiratory syndrome coronavirus 2 infection, COVID-19, with lower levels being associated with more severe clinical outcomes...Although total testosterone levels increased over time after COVID-19, more than 50% of men who recovered from the disease still had circulating testosterone levels suggestive for a condition of hypogonadism at 7-month follow-up. In as many as 10% of cases, testosterone levels even further decreased. Of clinical relevance, the higher the burden of comorbid conditions at presentation, the lower the probability of testosterone levels recovery over time.

https://pubmed.ncbi.nlm.nih.gov/34409772/

**Testosterone and Covid-19: An update**...There is overwhelming evidence to suggest that male gender is at a higher risk of developing more severe Covid-19 disease and thus having poorer clinical outcomes...the evidence so far suggests that the role of testosterone in Covid-19 is a double-edged sword, with some studies suggesting that a low testosterone state is protective in men in certain situations, yet increasing amounts of evidence suggests lower T in male patients is associated with increased Covid-19 severity and mortality. However, lack of evidence on the effect of pre-infection circulating T, contradictory reports on the effects of ADT on SAR-CoV-2 infection, and incomplete understanding of the underlying biological mechanisms makes it difficult to conclude if T is a marker or mediator of Covid-19 severity. Indeed, the mechanisms are likely to be multidimensional and influenced by a wide range of interacting factors that can be specific to the individual patient. Furthermore, the potential of TTh in men with Covid-19 to aid recovery and the effect of testosterone on long Covid are still to be extensively investigated.

https://www.ncbi.nlm.nih.gov/pmc/articles/PMC9537909/

**Role of testosterone in COVID-19 patients – A double-edged sword?**...COVID-19 affects males twice as frequently as females with significantly increased severity and mortality. Current data suggest a direct correlation between the lower level of serum testosterone, inflammatory cytokines, disease severity, and poor clinical outcomes among male patients with COVID-19. The gradual decline in total and free testosterone levels has a direct correlation with serious pulmonary complications requiring advanced care (ICU, ventilators, ECMO, etc.). SARS-CoV-2 utilizes Angiotensin-Converting Enzyme II (ACE2) for entry in the host cell, and Transmembrane Protease, Serine 2 (TMPRSS2) to prime spike protein of SARS-CoV-2. Testosterone induces ACE-2 expression, a critical pulmonary protective enzyme. Low testosterone levels in males have a direct correlation with the high probability of ICU admission and the worse disease outcome (ARDS, duration of ICU stay, mortality). On the contrary, however, high testosterone levels can lead to thrombosis which is also one of the fatal manifestations in COVID-19 patients. A critical evaluation of the serum testosterone and its relevance to COVID-19 is warranted to re-evaluate strategies to effectively triage, prioritize, and manage high-risk patients for ICU admission, survival outcomes, targeted solutions, and operational algorithms.

https://www.ncbi.nlm.nih.gov/pmc/articles/PMC7494488/

**Testosterone in males with COVID-19: a 12-month cohort study**...Male patients with COVID-19 have been found with reduced serum total testosterone (tT) levels and with more severe clinical outcomes...Circulating tT levels keep increasing over time in men after COVID-19. Still, almost 30% of men who recovered from COVID-19 had low circulating T levels suggestive for a condition of hypogonadism at a minimum 12-month follow-up.

https://pubmed.ncbi.nlm.nih.gov/36251583/

*"COVID-19 is known to depress testosterone levels in males."*

**Steven Magee**

## Fish Oil Supplements

**Potential of Omega 3 Supplementation for Coronavirus Disease 2019 (COVID-19): A Scoping Review**...COVID-19 can cause fever, cough, headache, and shortness of breath but patients with comorbidities can experience worsening and death. An action is needed to treat this condition in COVID-19 patients. Omega 3 fatty acids may be one possibility associated with COVID-19 prevention, management, and treatment...severe COVID-19 patients have low levels of omega 3 in their blood. Omega 3 was considered to reduce the risk of positive for SARS-CoV-infection and the duration of symptoms, overcome the renal and respiratory dysfunction, and increase survival rate in COVID 19 patients. Omega 3 fatty acid supplementations were thought to have a potential effect in preventing and treating COVID-19.

https://www.ncbi.nlm.nih.gov/pmc/articles/PMC9012318/

**Omega 3 Fatty Acids and COVID-19: A Comprehensive Review**...Patients diagnosed with COVID-19 present with symptoms ranging from none to severe and include fever, shortness of breath, dry cough, anosmia, and gastrointestinal abnormalities. Severe complications are largely due to overdrive of the host immune system leading to "cytokine storm". This results in disseminated intravascular coagulation, acute respiratory distress syndrome, multiple organ dysfunction syndrome, and death. Due to its highly infectious nature and concerning mortality rate, every effort has been focused on prevention and creating new medications or repurposing old treatment options to ameliorate the suffering of COVID-19 patients including the immune dysregulation. Omega-3 fatty acids are known to be incorporated throughout the body into the bi-phospholipid layer of the cell membrane leading to the production of less pro-inflammatory mediators compared to other fatty acids that are more prevalent in the Western diet. In this article, the benefits of omega-3 fatty acids, especially eicosapentaenoic acid and docosahexaenoic acid, including their anti-inflammatory, immunomodulating, and possible antiviral effects have been discussed.

https://www.ncbi.nlm.nih.gov/pmc/articles/PMC7779984/


**Long COVID and long chain fatty acids (LCFAs): Psychoneuroimmunity implication of omega-3 LCFAs in delayed consequences of COVID-19**...The global spread of severe acute respiratory syndrome coronavirus 2 (SARS-CoV-2) has led to the lasting pandemic of coronavirus disease 2019 (COVID-19) and the post-acute phase sequelae of heterogeneous negative impacts in multiple systems known as the "long COVID." The mechanisms of neuropsychiatric complications of long COVID are multifactorial, including long-term tissue damages from direct CNS viral involvement, unresolved systemic inflammation and oxidative stress, maladaptation of the renin-angiotensin-aldosterone system and coagulation system, dysregulated immunity, the dysfunction of neurotransmitters and hypothalamus–pituitaryadrenal (HPA) axis, and the psychosocial stress imposed by societal changes in response to this pandemic. The strength of safety, well-acceptance, and accumulating scientific evidence has now afforded nutritional medicine a place in the mainstream of neuropsychiatric intervention and prophylaxis. Long chain omega-3 polyunsaturated fatty acids (omega-3 or n-3 PUFAs) might have favorable effects on immunity, inflammation, oxidative stress and psychoneuroimmunity at different stages of SARS-CoV-2 infection. Omega-3 PUFAs, particularly EPA, have shown effects in treating mood and neurocognitive disorders by reducing pro-inflammatory cytokines, altering the HPA axis, and modulating neurotransmission via lipid rafts. In addition, omega-3 PUFAs and their metabolites, including specialized pro-resolvin mediators, accelerate the process of cleansing chronic inflammation and restoring tissue homeostasis, and therefore offer a promising strategy for Long COVID. In this article, we explore in a systematic review the putative molecular mechanisms by which omega-3 PUFAs and their metabolites counteract the negative effects of long COVID on the brain, behavior, and immunity.

https://www.ncbi.nlm.nih.gov/pmc/articles/PMC8977215/

**Bioactive omega-3 fatty acids are associated with reduced risk and severity of SARS-CoV-2 infection**...higher DHA status is associated with lower risk of testing positive for infection with SARS-CoV-2 and of being hospitalized with COVID-19. There is also an indication that higher DHA status is associated with reduced risk of mortality for COVID-19, although this effect was attenuated at the very highest status level. These findings suggest that consuming more long-chain omega-3 fatty acids (EPA and DHA) should be encouraged as a strategy to reduce the impact of the ongoing SARS-CoV-2 pandemic and of future respiratory virus infection outbreaks. Increased intake of EPA and DHA can be achieved through consumption of fatty fish or use of supplements containing EPA and DHA.

https://www.ncbi.nlm.nih.gov/pmc/articles/PMC9972879/

*"Fish oil supplements appear to reduce the risks from COVID-19 infection."*

**Steven Magee**

## Live Culture Yogurt

**Theoretical benefits of yogurt-derived bioactive peptides and probiotics in COVID-19 patients – A narrative review and hypotheses**...observational studies suggested lower COVID-19 severity in populations consuming fermented foods, no controlled study investigated the role of diet. Yogurt, a fermented dairy product, exhibits interesting properties related to the presence of bioactive peptides and probiotics that may play a beneficial role in COVID-19 presentation and outcome. Peptides contained in yogurt are responsible for angiotensin-converting enzyme-inhibitory, bradykinin potentiating, antiviral, anti-inflammatory, antithrombotic, and antioxidant effects. The types and activity of these peptides vary widely depending on their amino acid sequence, on the probiotics used in yogurt production and on intestinal digestion. Additionally, probiotics used in yogurt exhibit direct angiotensin-converting enzyme-inhibitory, antiviral and immune boosting activities. Since COVID-19 pathogenesis involves angiotensin II accumulation and bradykinin deficiency, yogurt bioactive peptides appear as potentially beneficial.

https://www.ncbi.nlm.nih.gov/pmc/articles/PMC8213517/

**Effects of yogurt containing probiotics on respiratory virus infections: Influenza H1N1 and SARS-CoV-2**...In a situation in which no established drug or treatment exists, consumption of proper food might be beneficial in maintaining health against external infections. We studied the potential effects of mixtures of probiotic strains on various viral infections. The purpose of this study was to assess the ability of yogurt containing probiotics to reduce the risk of respiratory viruses such as influenza H1N1 and SARS-CoV-2 infection. First, we performed in vitro tests using infected Madin-Darby canine kidney (MDCK) and Vero E6 cells, to evaluate the potential effects of yogurt containing high-dose probiotics against influenza H1N1 and SARS-CoV-2 infection. The yogurt significantly reduced plaque formation in the virus-infected cells. We also performed in vivo tests using influenza H1N1-infected C57BL/6 mice and SARS-CoV-2-infected Syrian golden hamsters, to evaluate the potential effects of yogurt. Yogurt was administered orally once daily during the experimental period. Yogurt was also administered orally as pretreatment once daily for 3 wk before viral infection. Regarding influenza H1N1, it was found that yogurt caused an increase in the survival rate, body weight, and IFN-γ, IgG1, and IL-10 levels against viral infection and a decrease in the inflammatory cytokines TNF-α and IL-6. Although the SARS-CoV-2 copy number was not significantly reduced in the lungs of yogurt-treated SARS-CoV-2-infected hamsters, the body weights and histopathological findings of the lungs were improved in the yogurt-treated group. In conclusion, we suggest that consumption of yogurt containing probiotics can lead to beneficial effects to prevent respiratory viral infections.

https://www.ncbi.nlm.nih.gov/pmc/articles/PMC9829060/

**The effect of probiotics on respiratory tract infection with special emphasis on COVID-19: Systemic review 2010–20...**To evaluate the effects of probiotics on respiratory tract infection (RTI) a systematic review of randomized controlled trials (RCTs) from January 2010 to January 2020 was conducted. The PubMed, Google Scholar, Embase, Scopus, Clinicaltrials.gov, and International Clinical Trials Registry Platform databases were systematically searched for the following keywords: respiratory tract infection, probiotics, viral infection, COVID-19, and clinical trial. A total of 27 clinical trials conducted on 9433 patients with RTI plus 10 ongoing clinical studies of probiotics intervention in Coronavirus disease 2019 (COVID-19) were reviewed. The review looked at the potency of probiotics for the hindrance and/or treatment of RTI diseases, this may also apply to COVID-19. The review found that probiotics could significantly increase the plasma levels of cytokines, the effect of influenza vaccine and quality of life, as well as reducing the titer of viruses and the incidence and duration of respiratory infections. These antiviral and immune-modulating activities and their ability to stimulate interferon production recommend the use of probiotics as an adjunctive therapy to prevent COVID-19.  Based on this extensive review of RCTs we suggest that probiotics are a rational complementary treatment for RTI diseases and a viable option to support faster recovery.

https://www.ncbi.nlm.nih.gov/pmc/articles/PMC7871912/

**Kefir: A protective dietary supplementation against viral infection**...'Kefir' is a fermented milk drink similar to a thin yogurt that is made from kefir grains. Kefir and its probiotic contents can modulate the immune system to suppress infections from viruses (e.g., Zika, hepatitis C, influenza, rotaviruses). The antiviral mechanisms of kefir involve enhancement of macrophage production, increasing phagocytosis, boosting production of cluster of differentiation-positive (CD4+), CD8+, immunoglobulin (Ig)G+ and IgA+ B cells, T cells, neutrophils, as well as cytokines (e.g., interleukin (IL)-2, IL-12, interferon gamma-$\gamma$). Kefir can act as an anti-inflammatory agent by reducing expression of IL-6, IL-1, TNF-$\alpha$, and interferon-$\gamma$. Hence, kefir might be a significant inhibitor of the 'cytokine storm' that contributes to COVID-19. Here, we review several studies with a particular emphasis on the effect of kefir consumption and their microbial composition against viral infection, as well as discussing the further development of kefir as a protective supplementary dietary against SARS-CoV-2 infection via modulating the immune response.

https://www.ncbi.nlm.nih.gov/pmc/articles/PMC7655491/

*"Live culture yogurt may speed up recovery from COVID-19."*

**Steven Magee**

## Amino Acids

**Evaluation of amino acid profile in serum of patients with Covid-19 for providing a new treatment strategy**...The present study shows that alterations not only one serum amino acids lenel but serveral amino acids may be of prognostic value in course of COVID-19 disease and they play an important role in its pathogenesis. It could also be suggested that the obtained data can be used as a biomarkers-treatment target in terms of the diagnosis of the disease, the course of the disease, and the effectiveness of the treatment. Specifically, the determination of amino acid profiles in patients with COVID-19 may be significant for developing different treatment strategies. Since there is not enough information about how the serum profile of amino acids is affected in SARS-CoV-2 disease, there is a need for new studies focusing on the serum amino acid profile. To better understand the disease, the present study results specifically recommend more studies to be planned to investigate the relationship between amino acids level and the immune system and further provide treatment strategies.

https://www.ncbi.nlm.nih.gov/pmc/articles/PMC9618340/

**Disturbed lipid and amino acid metabolisms in COVID-19 patients**...We performed targeted metabolomics covering up to 630 metabolites within several key metabolic pathways in plasma samples of 20 hospitalized COVID-19 patients and 37 matched controls. Plasma metabolic signatures specifically differentiated severe COVID-19 from control patients. The identified metabolic signatures indicated distinct alterations in both lipid and amino acid metabolisms in COVID-19 compared to control patient plasma. Systems biology-based analyses identified sphingolipid, tryptophan, tyrosine, glutamine, arginine, and arachidonic acid metabolism as mostly impacted pathways in COVID-19 patients. Notably, gamma-aminobutyric acid (GABA) was significantly reduced in COVID-19 patients and GABA plasma levels allowed for stratification of COVID-19 patients with high sensitivity and specificity. The data reveal large metabolic disturbances in COVID-19 patients and suggest use of GABA as potential biomarker and therapeutic target for the infection.

https://www.ncbi.nlm.nih.gov/pmc/articles/PMC8783191/


**Association between Circulating Amino Acids and COVID-19 Severity**...The severity of the symptoms associated with COVID-19 is highly variable, and has been associated with circulating amino acids as a group of analytes in metabolomic studies. However, for each individual amino acid, there are discordant results among studies. The aims of the present study were: (i) to investigate the association between COVID-19-symptom severity and circulating amino-acid concentrations; and (ii) to assess the ability of circulating amino-acid levels to predict adverse outcomes (intensive-care-unit admission or hospital death). We studied a sample of 736 participants from the Biobanque Québécoise COVID-19. All participants tested positive for COVID-19, and the severity of symptoms was determined using the World-Health-Organization criteria. Circulating amino acids were measured by HPLC-MS/MS. We used logistic models to assess the association between circulating amino acids concentrations and the odds of presenting mild vs. severe or mild vs. moderate symptoms, as well as their accuracy in predicting adverse outcomes. Patients with severe COVID-19 symptoms were older on average, and they had a higher prevalence of obesity and type 2 diabetes. Out of 20 amino acids tested, 16 were significantly associated with disease severity, with phenylalanine (positively) and cysteine (inversely) showing the strongest associations. These associations remained significant after adjustment for age, sex and body mass index. Phenylalanine had a fair ability to predict the occurrence of adverse outcomes, similar to traditionally measured laboratory variables. A multivariate model including both circulating amino acids and clinical variables had a 90% accuracy at predicting adverse outcomes in this sample. In conclusion, patients presenting severe COVID-19 symptoms have an altered amino-acid profile, compared to those with mild or moderate symptoms.

https://pubmed.ncbi.nlm.nih.gov/36837819/

**The Central Role of Clinical Nutrition in COVID-19 Patients During and After Hospitalization in Intensive Care Unit**...The COVID-19-positive patient who is subject to a hyperinflammatory condition associated with lung injury with the development of pneumonia is hospitalized in the intensive care unit. Before resolving and overcoming the "cytokine storm," with overexpression of pro-inflammatory interleukins (IL-, Il-6), this patient will be intubated for more than 48 h and therefore needs adequate nutrition. Malnutrition can lead to sarcopenia with a decrease in lean body mass and worsening of the inflammatory state underway. In addition, severe debilitation, if not corrected with adequate nutrition, can greatly lengthen rehabilitation times with prolonged hospitalization, increased costs, and reduced turn over already in crisis due to the health emergency caused by coronavirus. The aim of this study is to focus attention on the nutritional importance that must be provided in case of COVID-19 together with pharmacological treatments to lower the number of circulating proinflammatory cytokines. Oral, enteral, and parenteral nutrition should always be carried out according to the patient's condition and, in the case of a hyperinflammatory patient, such as the one affected by COVID-19, it has been shown that the supplementation of amino acids helps to lower the inflammatory state and promotes normal physiological recovery.

https://www.ncbi.nlm.nih.gov/pmc/articles/PMC7360691/

**L-amino-acids as immunity booster against COVID-19: DFT, molecular docking and MD simulations**...There is great interest to explore the importance of different amino-acids on immunity of human. Immunity helps to protect us from the pathogenic infections. The amino-acids are being use to give energy and is also used as an important basic molecule for the making of cells, protecting cell and others. Still, a little information is known for their importance in the inhibition of main protease of SARS-CoV-2. As known, tens of billions of humans are infected due to the SARS-CoV-2 and about a million of deaths are reported due to it or COVID. As of now, no promising drug is available in the market to cure the patients from this infection. Even, the medicines beings used for the partial cure may have some side effects. Therefore, the focus is to explore the natural amino-acids against the Mpro of SARS-CoV-2 as using of amino-acids is not toxic to humans. In the present work, authors have studied the amino-acids using DFT calculations and then they were explored for their promising role in the inhibition of main protease of SARS-CoV-2 using molecular docking and molecular dynamics simulations. Out of the 20 amino-acids, arginine found to best against the main protease of SARS-CoV-2 using the molecular docking and the binding energy was -0.94 kcal/ mol. Further, molecular dynamics simulations for the main protease of SARS-CoV-2 with and without arginine was performed using the Amber and different thermodynamic parameters like $\Delta H$ and $T\Delta S$ to get $\Delta G$, comes out to be 2.74 kcal/mol. It is expected that arginine can boost the immunity.

https://www.ncbi.nlm.nih.gov/pmc/articles/PMC8590830/

*"COVID-19 is known to disturb the amino acid systems of the human body."*

**Steven Magee**

## Glycine

**Can glycine mitigate COVID-19 associated tissue damage and cytokine storm ?**...Because of its excellent safety record, promising anti-inflammatory properties, and wide availability and affordability, I propose that clinical trials with glycine as a mitigator of cytokine storms should be conducted as soon as possible in COVID-19 patients. It may be administered either orally in patients with moderate symptoms or intravenously in patients with severe symptoms at doses of 0.5-1.0 g/kg/d. In early stages of the disease, glycine may suppress or blunt the onset of virus-induced cytokine storm. In late stages of the disease, its cytoprotective effect may protect lung tissues from severe damage and ARDS, the leading cause of the mortality. Under these circumstances, it may be used in conjunction with other treatments, such as dexamethasone, which was shown to reduce cell death in advanced stage patients; or radiotherapy, as reported recently; or anti-viral agents, such as remdesivir. It is likely that glycine may enhance the therapeutic effects of those treatments.

https://www.ncbi.nlm.nih.gov/pmc/articles/PMC7574884/

**D,L-Lysine-Acetylsalicylate + Glycine (LASAG) Reduces SARS-CoV-2 Replication and Shows an Additive Effect with Remdesivir**...Using mono cell culture systems and a more complex chip model, we investigated the effects of the acetylsalicylic acid (ASA) salt D, L-lysine-acetylsalicylate + glycine (LASAG) on SARS-CoV-2 infection in vitro. ASA is commonly known as Aspirin® and is one of the most frequently used medications worldwide. Our data indicate an inhibitory effect of LASAG on SARS-CoV-2 replication and SARS-CoV-2-induced expression of pro-inflammatory cytokines and coagulation factors. Remarkably, our data point to an additive effect of the combination of LASAG and the antiviral acting drug remdesivir on SARS-CoV-2 replication in vitro.

https://www.ncbi.nlm.nih.gov/pmc/articles/PMC9266999/

**Severe Glutathione Deficiency, Oxidative Stress and Oxidant Damage in Adults Hospitalized with COVID-19: Implications for GlyNAC (Glycine and N-Acetylcysteine) Supplementation**...Oxidative stress (OxS) is a harmful condition caused by excess reactive-oxygen species (ROS) and is normally neutralized by antioxidants among which Glutathione (GSH) is the most abundant. GSH deficiency results in amplified OxS due to compromised antioxidant defenses. Because little is known about GSH or OxS in COVID-19 infection, we measured GSH, TBARS (a marker of OxS) and F2-isoprostane (marker of oxidant damage) concentrations in 60 adult patients hospitalized with COVID-19. Compared to uninfected controls, COVID-19 patients of all age groups had severe GSH deficiency, increased OxS and elevated oxidant damage which worsened with advancing age. These defects were also present in younger age groups, where they do not normally occur. Because GlyNAC (combination of glycine and N-acetylcysteine) supplementation has been shown in clinical trials to rapidly improve GSH deficiency, OxS and oxidant damage, GlyNAC supplementation has implications for combating these defects in COVID-19 infected patients and warrants urgent investigation.

https://www.ncbi.nlm.nih.gov/pmc/articles/PMC8773164/

**Anti-inflammatory activity of ivermectin in late-stage COVID-19 may reflect activation of systemic glycine receptors**...Ivermectin, a drug commonly used to treat a range of parasitic infections, has been shown to halve the mortality elicited by a fatal dose of lipopolysaccharide in mice, in an oral dose (4 mg/kg) that can be extrapolated to 2–4 times the standard clinical dose in humans (0.2 mg/kg). It has been suggested that this phenomenon is highly pertinent to the clinical utility of ivermectin in the cytokine storm phase of COVID-19, which has been documented in a number of clinical studies. A meta-analysis of 18 clinical studies to date examining the impact of ivermectin therapy in hospitalised COVID-19 patients has observed a roughly 68% reduction in mortality associated with its usage. The basis of ivermectin's potent anti-inflammatory activity remains unclear. However, it is notable that ivermectin can act as a partial agonist for glycine-gated strychnine-inhibitable chloride channels, which are expressed by a number of types of immune cells—including alveolar macrophages and neutrophils—as well as vascular endothelium. The anti-inflammatory effects of high-dose dietary glycine in rodents have been attributed to activation of such channels on immune and endothelial cells. The mechanism whereby glycine receptor activation achieves these effects remains unclear; hyperpolarisation of plasma membranes may be involved, as well as inhibition of endosomal nicotinamide adenine dinucleotide phosphat oxidase activity. In striking homology to the effects of ivermectin, high dietary glycine (5% of diet) has been shown to halve the mortality of a lethal dose of lipopolysaccharide (LPS) in rats. Glycine preadministration also blunts the lung injury induced by inhalation of aerosolised LPS in mice; this effect is associated with inhibition of NLR family pyrin domain containing 3 (NLRP3) inflammasome activation (thought to play a key role in COVID-19 lung inflammation and production of proinflammatory cytokines). Moreover, it is notable that, whereas 1 mM ivermectin suppresses the activating effect of LPS on Kupffer cells in vitro, removal of chloride from the medium completely eliminates ivermectin's impact in this regard. Nonetheless, it is not completely straightforward to predict that ivermectin administration will activate glycine-gated chloride receptors in vivo. At a concentration of 0.03 µM, ivermectin does not directly activate such receptors, but rather potentiates their response to sub-saturating concentrations of glycine. As ivermectin increases to 0.3 µM, these receptors are irreversibly activated by ivermectin, and glycine cannot further activate them. However, since ivermectin is only a partial agonist, the maximal channel activity achieved with ivermectin is about 20% less than that seen with a saturating concentration of glycine. The lung concentration of ivermectin achieved after a single standard dose (0.2 mg/kg) is estimated to be around 0.09 µM. The affinity of glycine for the homomeric alpha1 glycine receptor has been determined to be about 160 µM, whereas human fasting plasma glycine concentrations are near 200 μM. These values appear consistent with the possibility that clinical concentrations of ivermectin could indeed boost the activity of systemic—as opposed to central nervous system—glycine receptors in humans. (Ivermectin is largely excluded from the brain by P-glycoprotein transporters, which accounts for its relative safety.) It is therefore suggested that the clinical utility of ivermectin in the cytokine storm phase of COVID-19 reflects, at least in part, an anti-inflammatory effect mediated by increased activation of glycine receptors on leukocytes and possibly vascular endothelium. An evident corollary of this is that ingestion of high-dose glycine may provide somewhat analogous anti-inflammatory protection in COVID-19, as has previously been suggested. However, in light of accumulating evidence that ivermectin may have important utility for the primary prevention of COVID-19, it is likely that it also exerts an antiviral effect with respect to SARS-CoV-2, as suggested by in vitro studies. It is not clear whether glycine receptor agonism might have anything to do with this effect.

https://www.ncbi.nlm.nih.gov/pmc/articles/PMC8057070/

*"Glycine combined with carnitine significantly reduced hypoxic altitude sickness symptoms in me."*

**Steven Magee**

## L-Carnitine

**Effects of L-carnitine supplementation in patients with mild-to-moderate COVID-19 disease: a pilot study**...The control group received their standard hospital treatment only. In addition to standard medications, the intervention group received 3000 mg oral L-carnitine daily in three divided doses for five days...Higher means of O2 saturation were observed in the intervention rather than in the control group. Mean erythrocyte sedimentation rate (ESR) and C-reactive protein (CRP) were significantly lower in the intervention group. Furthermore, mean alkaline phosphatase (ALP) activity and lactate dehydrogenase (LDH) were lower in the intervention group. Also, lower mean serum creatine phosphokinase (CPK) was observed in the intervention group. No significant differences were observed in terms of clinical symptoms; however, six patients (14%) in the control group died due to the complications of COVID-19, while all patients in the intervention group survived...L-carnitine can be considered as a drug supplement in patients with COVID-19.

https://www.ncbi.nlm.nih.gov/pmc/articles/PMC9395946/

**Can l-carnitine reduce post-COVID-19 fatigue?**...A significant number of patients infected with the new coronavirus suffer from chronic fatigue syndrome after COVID-19, and their symptoms may persist for months after the infection. Nevertheless, no particular treatment for post-disease fatigue has been found. At the same time, many clinical trials have shown the effectiveness of l-carnitine in relieving fatigue caused by the treatment of diseases such as cancer, MS, and many other diseases. Therefore, it can be considered as a potential option to eliminate the effects of fatigue caused by COVID-19, and its consumption is recommended in future clinical trials to evaluate its effectiveness and safety.

https://www.ncbi.nlm.nih.gov/pmc/articles/PMC8667465/

**Carnitine and COVID-19 Susceptibility and Severity: A Mendelian Randomization Study**...Recent studies have proposed the potential role of carnitine as therapy options for COVID-19, but whether there is any correlation between them has not been explored yet. Meanwhile, unmeasured confounding factors in clinical studies can potentially bias the association evidence, as is a common criticism inherent to observational studies. Here, based on results from comprehensive two-sample MR analyses, we demonstrated that higher carnitine level was causally associated with decreased susceptibility and severity of COVID-19. Carnitine occurs in two forms known as D-carnitine and L-carnitine, and only L-carnitine is biologically active in the body. L-carnitine is an essential carrier for long-chain fatty acids from the cytosol through the inner mitochondrial membrane into the matrix, where β-oxidation takes place. Although no studies have investigated the correlation between carnitine and COVID-19, previous research on carnitine might provide some insights from molecular aspects of why L-carnitine might protect against COVID-19. L-carnitine plays an important role in fatty acid metabolism and could act as an adjuvant agent in the improvement of dyslipidemia. L-carnitine was previously found to increase high-density lipoprotein and lower triglyceride, total cholesterol and low-density cholesterol, while dyslipidemia has been shown to be associated with the risk and severity of COVID-19 repeatedly. In addition, as an effective antioxidant, L-carnitine was involved in modulating the mechanisms of the immune system and the nervous system, and could inhibit the expression of inflammatory factors. Antioxidants supplementation has been recommended in therapeutic strategies against COVID-19, since antioxidant therapy could improve oxygenation rates, glutathione levels and strengthen the immune response. Meanwhile, anti-inflammatory drugs were suggested to potentially inhibit a key enzyme in the replication and transcription of SARS-CoV-2, and anti-inflammatory agents have also been proposed as potential therapies for COVID-19 due to their prevention of cardiovascular events. Furthermore, L-carnitine plays a critical role in energy production, as it transports long-chain fatty acids into the mitochondria so they can be oxidized to produce energy. More energy for the immune system means more immune cells can be produced to protect against infection from virus. Lastly, current evidence showed that severely ill patients with COVID-19 tend to have a high concentration of pro-inflammatory cytokines, such as IL-6, compared to those who are moderately ill, and the high level of cytokines also indicates a poor prognosis in COVID-19. L-carnitine could suppress the production of pro-inflammatory cytokines by preventing the hyperosmolarity-induced oxidative stress, and thus might help prevent patients with COVID-19 from cytokine storm. Taken together, so many biological functions make L-carnitine a potential therapeutic option to protect against COVID-19. Unfortunately, no clinical or epidemiological studies have investigated the correlation between them. Here, using the MR approach, we clarified the protective role of carnitine on COVID-19 susceptibility and severity from a genetic perspective. Future clinical or functional studies could put importance to this, and further explore the role of carnitine in protecting against COVID-19.

https://www.ncbi.nlm.nih.gov/pmc/articles/PMC8656944/


**Dietary supplements for the management of COVID-19 symptoms...**The aim of this paper is to review the relationship between COVID-19 and nutrition and to discuss to most up-to-date dietary supplements proposed for COVID-19 treatment and prevention. Nutrition and nutritional dysregulations, such as obesity and malnutrition, are prominent risk factors for severe COVID-19. These factors exert anti-inflammatory and proinflammatory effects on the immune system, thus exacerbating or reducing the immunological response against the virus. As for the nutritional habits, the Western diet induces a chronic inflammatory state, whereas the Mediterranean diet exerts anti-inflammatory effects and has been proposed for ameliorating COVID-19 evolution and symptoms. Several vaccines have been researched and commercialized for COVID-19 prevention, whereas several drugs, although clinically tested, have not shown promising effects. To compensate for the lack of treatment, several supplements have been recommended for preventing or ameliorating COVID-19 symptoms. Thus, it is critical to review the dietary supplements proposed for COVID-19 treatment. Supplements containing α-cyclodextrin and hydroxytyrosol exhibited promising effects in several clinical trials and reduced the severity of the outcomes and the duration of the infection. Moreover, a supplement containing hydroxytyrosol, acetyl L-carnitine, and vitamins B, C, and D improved the symptoms of patients with post-COVID syndrome.

https://www.ncbi.nlm.nih.gov/pmc/articles/PMC9710408/

*"L-Carnitine works with glycine to significantly reduce hypoxic altitude sickness in me."*

**Steven Magee**

## L-Carnitine L-Tartrate

**L-Carnitine Tartrate Downregulates the ACE2 Receptor and Limits SARS-CoV-2 Infection**...In this study, we show that L-carnitine tartrate supplementation in humans and rodents led to significant decreases of key host dependency factors, notably angiotensin-converting enzyme 2 (ACE2), transmembrane protease serine 2 (TMPRSS2), and Furin, which are responsible for viral attachment, viral spike S-protein cleavage, and priming for viral fusion and entry. Interestingly, pre-treatment of Calu-3, human lung epithelial cells, with L-carnitine tartrate led to a significant and dose-dependent inhibition of the infection by SARS-CoV-2. Infection inhibition coincided with a significant decrease in ACE2 mRNA expression levels. These data suggest that L-carnitine tartrate should be tested with appropriate trials in humans for the possibility to limit SARS-CoV-2 infection.

https://pubmed.ncbi.nlm.nih.gov/33919991/

**Combined Metabolic Activators Accelerates Recovery in Mild-to-Moderate COVID-19**...COVID-19 is associated with mitochondrial dysfunction and metabolic abnormalities, including the deficiencies in nicotinamide adenine dinucleotide (NAD+) and glutathione metabolism. Here it is investigated if administration of a mixture of combined metabolic activators (CMAs) consisting of glutathione and NAD+ precursors can restore metabolic function and thus aid the recovery of COVID-19 patients. CMAs include l-serine, N-acetyl-l-cysteine, nicotinamide riboside, and l-carnitine tartrate, salt form of l-carnitine. Placebo-controlled, open-label phase 2 study and double-blinded phase 3 clinical trials are conducted to investigate the time of symptom-free recovery on ambulatory patients using CMAs. The results of both studies show that the time to complete recovery is significantly shorter in the CMA group (6.6 vs 9.3 d) in phase 2 and (5.7 vs 9.2 d) in phase 3 trials compared to placebo group. A comprehensive analysis of the plasma metabolome and proteome reveals major metabolic changes. Plasma levels of proteins and metabolites associated with inflammation and antioxidant metabolism are significantly improved in patients treated with CMAs as compared to placebo. The results show that treating patients infected with COVID-19 with CMAs lead to a more rapid symptom-free recovery, suggesting a role for such a therapeutic regime in the treatment of infections leading to respiratory problems.

https://www.ncbi.nlm.nih.gov/pmc/articles/PMC8420376/

### *"L-Carnitine L-Tartrate appears to limit the COVID-19 infection."*

**Steven Magee**

# GPLC

**Glycine propionyl l-carnitine attenuates d-Galactosamine induced fulminant hepatic failure in wistar rats**...Glycine propionyl l-carnitine (GPLC) is a propionyl ester of carnitine that includes an additional glycine component. The present study evaluated hepatoprotective effect of GPLC in d-Galactosamine (d-GalN) induced fulminant hepatic failure. Rats were intraperitonially administered d-GalN (700mg/kgBW). GPLC was given as a pre-treatment (35mg/kgBW/day) for 1month followed by a single dose of d-GalN on the 31st day. d-GalN administration resulted in increased mortality and serum ALT and AST activities. These increases were significantly attenuated by GPLC. d-GalN treatment increased hepatic lipid peroxidation and a decrease in reduced glutathione content was observed. GPLC pre-treatment significantly decreased lipid peroxidation and augmented the level of GSH. d-GalN increased the circulating level of TNF-α and ATM-Kinase and MAP-Kinase expression. GPLC supplementation inhibited the increase in serum TNF-α and ATM-Kinase and MAP-Kinase expression. d-GalN treatment increased the level of Bax and Caspase-3 m-RNA while as a decline was observed in Bcl2 m-RNA. GPLC prevented the increase in Caspase-3 and Bax m-RNA and at the same time augmented the expression of Bcl2 m-RNA. Our findings suggest that GPLC alleviates d-GalN induced liver injury by strengthening antioxidative defense system and reducing apoptotic signalling pathways.

https://pubmed.ncbi.nlm.nih.gov/24565947/

*"GPLC is the only supplement that will significantly reduce my hypoxic altitude sickness on its own."*

**Steven Magee**

# L-Arginine

**l-Arginine and COVID-19: An Update**...l-Arginine is involved in many different biological processes and recent reports indicate that it could also play a crucial role in the coronavirus disease 2019 (COVID-19), caused by the severe acute respiratory syndrome coronavirus 2 (SARS-CoV-2)...The functional contribution of l-Arginine in many biological processes is extremely significant, especially in the control of endothelial and immune activities. There is a strong rationale indicating a beneficial effect of l-Arginine in COVID-19, and preliminary results from a randomized clinical trial seem to support this view.

https://www.ncbi.nlm.nih.gov/pmc/articles/PMC8619186/

**Combining l-Arginine with vitamin C improves long-COVID symptoms: The LINCOLN Survey**...Our survey indicates that the supplementation with l-Arginine + Vitamin C has beneficial effects in Long-COVID, in terms of attenuating its typical symptoms and improving effort perception.

https://www.ncbi.nlm.nih.gov/pmc/articles/PMC9295384/

**Targeting Arginine in COVID-19-Induced Immunopathology and Vasculopathy**...Emerging data have identified a deficiency of circulating arginine in patients with COVID-19. Arginine is a semi-essential amino acid that serves as key regulator of immune and vascular cell function. Arginine is metabolized by nitric oxide (NO) synthase to NO which plays a pivotal role in host defense and vascular health, whereas the catabolism of arginine by arginase to ornithine contributes to immune suppression and vascular disease. Notably, arginase activity is upregulated in COVID-19 patients in a disease-dependent fashion, favoring the production of ornithine and its metabolites from arginine over the synthesis of NO. This rewiring of arginine metabolism in COVID-19 promotes immune and endothelial cell dysfunction, vascular smooth muscle cell proliferation and migration, inflammation, vasoconstriction, thrombosis, and arterial thickening, fibrosis, and stiffening, which can lead to vascular occlusion, muti-organ failure, and death. Strategies that restore the plasma concentration of arginine, inhibit arginase activity, and/or enhance the bioavailability and potency of NO represent promising therapeutic approaches that may preserve immune function and prevent the development of severe vascular disease in patients with COVID-19…Emerging clinical studies have identified abnormalities in the metabolism of arginine in COVID-19 patients that results in a lower circulating level of this amino acid. Moreover, there is an increase in ARG1 expression with COVID-19 that shifts the metabolism of arginine away from the synthesis of NO towards the formation of ornithine, polyamines, and proline. This maladaptive response in arginine metabolism may contribute to COVID-19-mediated impairments in immune and vascular function. Strategies that target the loss of plasma arginine and the reprogramming of arginine metabolism and increase the bioavailability and potency of NO in COVID-19 provide promising approaches in mitigating the devastating consequences of SARS-CoV-2 infection.

https://www.ncbi.nlm.nih.gov/pmc/articles/PMC8953281/

**COVID-19 and L-arginine Supplementations: Yet to Find the Missed Key**…Current coronavirus disease (COVID-19) is regarded as a primary respiratory and vascular disease leading to acute lung injury (ALI), acute respiratory distress syndrome (ARDS), and endothelial dysfunction (ED) in severe cases. The causative virus of COVID-19 is SARS-CoV-2, which binds angiotensin-converting enzyme 2 (ACE2) for its entry. It has been shown that ED is linked to various COVID-19 complications since endothelial cells are regarded as the chief barrier against SARS-CoV- 2 invasion. SARS-CoV-2-indued ED leads to endotheliitis and thrombosis due to endothelial nitric oxide (NO) inhibition with subsequent vasoconstriction and tissue hypoxia. Loss of vasodilator NO and anti-thrombin factor from endothelial SARS-CoV-2 infection contribute to the progression of vascular dysfunction and coagulopathy. Therefore, NO restoration improves pulmonary function and hinders viral replication during respiratory viral infections, including COVID-19. L-arginine is a semiessential amino acid that has antiviral and immunomodulatory effects as well as improves the biosynthesis of NO in endothelial cells. L-arginine may reduce the risk of ALI through inhibition of generation of peroxynitrite and suppression of the release of proinflammatory cytokines from alveolar macrophages. Of interest, restoration of NO by L-arginine may attenuate SARS-CoV-2 infection through different mechanisms, including reduction binding of SARS-CoV-2 to ACE2, inhibition of transmembrane protease serine-type 2 (TMPRSS2), critical for the activation of SARS-CoV-2 spike protein and cellular entry, inhibition proliferation and replication of SARS-CoV-2, and prevention of SARS-CoV-2-induced coagulopathy. In conclusion, through antiviral and immunomodulatory effects, L-arginine and released NO have mutual and interrelated actions against SARS-CoV-2 infection.

https://pubmed.ncbi.nlm.nih.gov/35549865/

*"L-arginine boosts the nitric oxide content of the human body."*

**Steven Magee**

## <u>L-Citrulline</u>

**Patients with COVID-19 present with low plasma citrulline concentrations that associate with systemic inflammation and gastrointestinal symptoms**...a majority of patients with moderate to severe COVID-19 had decreased levels of plasma citrulline, which correlated with digestive symptoms and systemic inflammation. In addition to previous indirect evidence, our study suggests that enterocytes themselves may be affected by SARS-CoV-2, leading to gastrointestinal symptoms and worsening of systemic inflammation. Low citrulline is likely involved in SARS-CoV-2-associated diarrhea by causing alteration of intestinal permeability and enterocyte malabsorption. It could also participate in the significant weight loss that is observed in patients with COVID-19...Citrulline is very specific of total enterocyte mass, suggesting a direct impact of SARS-CoV-2 on the enterocytes. Intestinal ischemia, through hypoxic injury and microvascular coagulopathy induced by SARS-CoV-2, could also be considered as a mechanism of enterocytes dysfunction.

https://www.ncbi.nlm.nih.gov/pmc/articles/PMC7332957/

**Nitric oxide boosters as defensive agents against COVID-19 infection: an opinion**...the possible role of nitric oxide (NO) releasers in aiding the immune system of a human body against this dreadful pandemic disease...Watermelon is one of the best sources of citrulline, an amino acid that's converted to arginine and, ultimately to nitric oxide...Social distancing (physical distancing) alone can't help in halting the spread of covid-19 infection. Though prevention is better than cure, but human body has to always be ready to combat infections. At least a dietary routine could be modified to allow inclusion of those foods which can help in boosting immune system. The article hence describes the significant use of NO as immune-modulator and agent to attain relief from the infection severity including breathlessness and chest pain. Due to some distinctive NO-releasing differences among inorganic and organic species, attention must be paid towards the design of efficient NO-releasing compounds.

https://www.ncbi.nlm.nih.gov/pmc/articles/PMC7754890/


**The Effect of L-Citrulline Supplementation on Outcomes of Critically Ill Patients under Mechanical Ventilation; a Double-Blind Randomized Controlled Trial**...For critically ill and injured patients, amino acids are crucial for nutritional and metabolic support. Citrulline, which has gained attention recently, is included in these immune-nutrition (IMN) formulas, along with arginine, n-3 fatty acids, glutamine, antioxidants, and nucleic acids. As our knowledge of altered amino acid metabolism in such patients increases, it is crucial to develop more effective parenteral and enteral amino acid replacement products. Following trauma and surgery, arginine and citrulline levels appear to decrease in critically ill patients. Moreover, these amino acids are reversely correlated with levels of cytokines and inflammatory markers. A growing body of evidence shows that cytokines can contribute to the emergence of critical illness. Cytokines are strongly related to higher disease severity in these states, while the persistence in the spread of the cytokinesis is associated with improvement in multiple organ failure (MOF). Orally ingested L-citrulline can result in the biosynthesis of L-arginine and, L-citrulline, and also enhance arginine bioavailability in the circulation, which acts as a precursor for nitric oxide (NO) formation. NO level could regulate vasodilation, blood flow, and muscle oxygenation...L-citrulline supplementation decreased the serum levels of FBS, LDL-C, TC, and hs-CRP, duration of invasive ventilation, and SOFA score. On the other hand, serum LDH levels and days alive and ventilator-free days within 28 days after admission significantly increased with Lcitrulline supplementation.

https://www.ncbi.nlm.nih.gov/pmc/articles/PMC9807954/


**COVID-19 Metabolomic-Guided Amino Acid Therapy Protects from Inflammation and Disease Sequelae**...A metabolic disorder is a contributing factor to deaths from COVID-19. However, the underlying mechanism of metabolic dysfunction in COVID-19 patients and the potential interventions are not elucidated. Here targeted plasma metabolomic is performed, and the metabolite profiles among healthy controls, and asymptomatic, moderate, and severe COVID-19 patients are compared. Among the altered metabolites, arachidonic acid and linolenic acid pathway metabolites are profoundly up-regulated in COVID-19 patients. Arginine biosynthesis, alanine, aspartate, and glutamate metabolism pathways are significantly disturbed in asymptomatic patients. In the comparison of metabolite variances among the groups, higher levels of l-citrulline and l-glutamine are found in asymptomatic carriers and moderate or severe patients at the remission stage. Furthermore, l-citrulline and l-glutamine combination therapy is demonstrated to effectively protect mice from coronavirus infection and endotoxin-induced sepsis, and is observed to efficiently prevent the occurrence of pulmonary fibrosis and central nervous system damage. Collectively, the data reveal the metabolite profile of asymptomatic COVID-19 patients and propose a potential strategy for COVID-19 treatment.

https://pubmed.ncbi.nlm.nih.gov/36775870/

**"*Citrulline converts into arginine and nitric oxide in the human body.*"**

**Steven Magee**

## L-Lysine

**Effects of Basic Amino Acids and Their Derivatives on SARS-CoV-2 and Influenza-A Virus Infection**...Amino acids have been implicated with virus infection and replication. Here, we demonstrate the effects of two basic amino acids, arginine and lysine, and their ester derivatives on infection of two enveloped viruses, SARS-CoV-2, and influenza A virus. We found that lysine and its ester derivative can efficiently block infection of both viruses in vitro. Furthermore, the arginine ester derivative caused a significant boost in virus infection. Studies on their mechanism of action revealed that the compounds potentially disturb virus uncoating rather than virus attachment and endosomal acidification. Our findings suggest that lysine supplementation and the reduction of arginine-rich food intake can be considered as prophylactic and therapeutic regimens against these viruses while also providing a paradigm for the development of broad-spectrum antivirals.

https://www.ncbi.nlm.nih.gov/pmc/articles/PMC8310019/

**D,L-Lysine-Acetylsalicylate + Glycine (LASAG) Reduces SARS-CoV-2 Replication and Shows an Additive Effect with Remdesivir**...The severe acute respiratory syndrome coronavirus 2 (SARS-CoV-2) causing the coronavirus disease-19 (COVID-19) is still challenging healthcare systems and societies worldwide. While vaccines are available, therapeutic strategies are developing and need to be adapted to each patient. Many clinical approaches focus on the repurposing of approved therapeutics against other diseases. However, the efficacy of these compounds on viral infection or even harmful secondary effects in the context of SARS-CoV-2 infection are sparsely investigated. Similarly, adverse effects of commonly used therapeutics against lifestyle diseases have not been studied in detail. Using mono cell culture systems and a more complex chip model, we investigated the effects of the acetylsalicylic acid (ASA) salt D, L-lysine-acetylsalicylate + glycine (LASAG) on SARS-CoV-2 infection in vitro. ASA is commonly known as Aspirin® and is one of the most frequently used medications worldwide. Our data indicate an inhibitory effect of LASAG on SARS-CoV-2 replication and SARS-CoV-2-induced expression of pro-inflammatory cytokines and coagulation factors. Remarkably, our data point to an additive effect of the combination of LASAG and the antiviral acting drug remdesivir on SARS-CoV-2 replication in vitro.

https://www.ncbi.nlm.nih.gov/pmc/articles/PMC9266999/

**Blocking viral infections with lysine-based polymeric nanostructures: a critical review**...The outbreak of the Covid-19 pandemic due to the SARS-CoV-2 coronavirus has accelerated the search for innovative antivirals with possibly broad-spectrum efficacy. One of the possible strategies is to inhibit the replication of the virus by preventing or limiting its entry into the cells. Nanomaterials derived from lysine, an essential amino acid capable of forming homopeptides of different shapes and sizes through thermal polymerization, are an exciting antiviral option. In this review, we have critically compared the antiviral activities and mechanisms of action of lysine and its possible analogues in the form of linear, hyperbranched, dendrimer and nanoparticle polymers. The polycationic nature, as well as the structure of polylysine in its various forms, favours the electrostatic interaction with viruses by inhibiting their replication and endocytosis. In the case of lysine alone, the antiviral action is instead carried out inside the cell. The experimental results obtained so far show that the development of antivirals based on amino acids that inhibit the entry of viruses into cells represents a definite possibility for developing challenging solutions against present and future pandemics.

https://pubmed.ncbi.nlm.nih.gov/35297436/

**Lysine 164 is critical for SARS-CoV-2 Nsp1 inhibition of host gene expression**...Given that coronavirus nonstructural protein 1 (nsp1) is a good target for attenuated vaccines, it is of great significance to explore the detailed characteristics of SARS-CoV-2 nsp1. Here, we first confirmed that SARS-CoV-2 nsp1 had a conserved function similar to that of SARS-CoV nsp1 in inhibiting host-protein synthesis and showed greater inhibition efficiency, as revealed by ribopuromycylation and Renilla luciferase (Rluc) reporter assays. Specifically, bioinformatics and biochemical experiments showed that by interacting with 40S ribosomal subunit, the lysine located at amino acid 164 (K164) was the key residue that enabled SARS-CoV-2 nsp1 to suppress host gene expression. Furthermore, as an inhibitor of host-protein expression, SARS-CoV-2 nsp1 contributed to cell-cycle arrest in G0/G1 phase, which might provide a favourable environment for virus production. Taken together, this research uncovered the detailed mechanism by which SARS-CoV-2 nsp1 K164 inhibited host gene expression, laying the foundation for the development of attenuated vaccines based on nsp1 modification.

https://www.ncbi.nlm.nih.gov/pmc/articles/PMC8116783/


*"Lysine is an amino acid that has antiviral properties."*

**Steven Magee**

## Creatine

**Can creatine help in pulmonary rehabilitation after COVID-19?**...COVID-19 pneumonia patients who responded successfully to intensive care treatments and were able to be discharged from hospital appear to experience a prolonged recovery, demanding resolute inpatient and outpatient rehabilitation services. Those include predominantly physiotherapy, occupational therapy, and speech-language retraining, with respect to recovery of the respiratory system as well as mobility and function. The recent European Society for Clinical Nutrition and Metabolism (ESPEN) concise guidance on clinical nutrition in COVID-19 patients properly addressed nutritional intervention and therapy as an integral part of the approach to patients victim to SARS-CoV-2 infection in the ICU setting, in an internal medicine ward setting as well as in general healthcare but omitted to consider nutritional guidance for COVID-19 survivors. Besides other early and short-term rehabilitative interventions, the International Task Force of the European Respiratory Society recently itemized adequate nutrition among rehabilitation needs for COVID-19 survivors upon release from hospital. Among other candidates, dietary creatine might emerge as one of the key elements of nutritional support following COVID-19 respiratory distress due to its beneficial effects demonstrated during rehabilitation in various lung conditions. For instance, creatine supplementation augments functional recovery during pulmonary rehabilitation in patients with chronic obstructive pulmonary disease, but also ameliorates cystic fibrosis, stroke, and respiratory failure, acting as an anti-inflammatory and energy-boosting agent. Although no disease-specific guidelines exist at present, a conventional creatine dosage of 5 g per day administered over 4 weeks or more might be risk-free and sufficient to back up pulmonary rehabilitation in COVID. Creatine is inexpensive, widely available, and has a favorable safety profile, therefore being a suitable promising compound that could meet a growing need for nutritional help during pulmonary rehabilitation in post-COVID-19 world.

https://www.ncbi.nlm.nih.gov/pmc/articles/PMC7649915/

**Increased Creatine Kinase May Predict A Worse COVID-19 Outcome**...Early reports from Asia suggested that increased serum levels of the muscular enzyme creatine-(phospho)-kinase (CK/CPK) could be associated with a more severe prognosis in COVID-19. The aim of this single-center retrospective cohort study of 331 consecutive COVID-19 patients who were hospitalized during Italy's "first wave" was to verify this relationship, and to evaluate the role of possible confounding factors (age, body mass index, gender, and comorbidities). We subdivided our cohort in two groups, based on "severe" (n = 99) or "mild" (n = 232) outcomes. "Severe" disease is defined here as death and/or mechanical invasive ventilation, in contrast to "mild" patients, who were discharged alive with no need for invasive ventilation; this latter group could also include those patients who were treated with non-invasive ventilation. The CK levels at admission were higher in those subjects who later experienced more severe outcomes (median, 126; range, 10-1672 U/L, versus median, 82; range, 12-1499 U/L, p = 0.01), and hyperCKemia >200 U/L was associated with a worse prognosis. Regression analysis confirmed that increased CK acted as an independent predictor for a "severe" outcome. HyperCKemia was generally transient, returning to normal during hospitalization in the majority of both "severe" and "mild" patients. Although the direct infection of voluntary muscle is unproven, transient muscular dysfunction is common during the course of COVID-19. The influence of this novel coronavirus on voluntary muscle really needs to be clarified.

https://pubmed.ncbi.nlm.nih.gov/33923719/

**Diagnostic and Pharmacological Potency of Creatine in Post-Viral Fatigue Syndrome**...Post-viral fatigue syndrome (PVFS) is a widespread chronic neurological disease with no definite etiological factor(s), no actual diagnostic test, and no approved pharmacological treatment, therapy, or cure. Among other features, PVFS could be accompanied by various irregularities in creatine metabolism, perturbing either tissue levels of creatine in the brain, the rates of phosphocreatine resynthesis in the skeletal muscle, or the concentrations of the enzyme creatine kinase in the blood. Furthermore, supplemental creatine and related guanidino compounds appear to impact both patient- and clinician-reported outcomes in syndromes and maladies with chronic fatigue. This paper critically overviews the most common disturbances in creatine metabolism in various PVFS populations, summarizes human trials on dietary creatine and creatine analogs in the syndrome, and discusses new frontiers and open questions for using creatine in a post-COVID-19 world.

https://pubmed.ncbi.nlm.nih.gov/33557013/

**Role of Creatine Supplementation in Conditions Involving Mitochondrial Dysfunction: A Narrative Review**...Creatine monohydrate (CrM) is one of the most widely used nutritional supplements among active individuals and athletes to improve high-intensity exercise performance and training adaptations. However, research suggests that CrM supplementation may also serve as a therapeutic tool in the management of some chronic and traumatic diseases. Creatine supplementation has been reported to improve high-energy phosphate availability as well as have antioxidative, neuroprotective, anti-lactatic, and calcium-homoeostatic effects. These characteristics may have a direct impact on mitochondrion's survival and health particularly during stressful conditions such as ischemia and injury. This narrative review discusses current scientific evidence for use or supplemental CrM as a therapeutic agent during conditions associated with mitochondrial dysfunction. Based on this analysis, it appears that CrM supplementation may have a role in improving cellular bioenergetics in several mitochondrial dysfunction-related diseases, ischemic conditions, and injury pathology and thereby could provide therapeutic benefit in the management of these conditions. However, larger clinical trials are needed to explore these potential therapeutic applications before definitive conclusions can be drawn.

https://www.ncbi.nlm.nih.gov/pmc/articles/PMC8838971/

*"Creatine has been used to treat hypoxic altitude sickness for many years."*

**Steven Magee**

## Enzymes

**Enzymes in the time of COVID-19: An overview about the effects in the human body, enzyme market, and perspectives for new drugs**...The rising pandemic caused by a coronavirus, resulted in a scientific quest to discover some effective treatments against its etiologic agent, the severe acute respiratory syndrome-coronavirus 2 (SARS-CoV-2). This research represented a significant scientific landmark and resulted in many medical advances. However, efforts to understand the viral mechanism of action and how the human body machinery is subverted during the infection are still ongoing. Herein, we contributed to this field with this compilation of the roles of both viral and human enzymes in the context of SARS-CoV-2 infection. In this sense, this overview reports that proteases are vital for the infection to take place: from SARS-CoV-2 perspective, the main protease (Mpro) and papain-like protease (PLpro) are highlighted; from the human body, angiotensin-converting enzyme-2, transmembrane serine protease-2, and cathepsins (CatB/L) are pointed out. In addition, the influence of the virus on other enzymes is reported as the JAK/STAT pathway and the levels of lipase, enzymes from the cholesterol metabolism pathway, amylase, aspartate aminotransferase, alanine aminotransferase, lactate dehydrogenase, and glyceraldehyde 3-phosphate dehydrogenase are also be disturbed in SARS-CoV-2 infection. Finally, this paper discusses the importance of detailed enzymatic studies for future treatments against SARS-CoV-2, and how some issues related to the syndrome treatment can create opportunities in the biotechnological market of enzymes and the development of new drugs.

https://www.ncbi.nlm.nih.gov/pmc/articles/PMC9350392/

**Role of proteolytic enzymes in the COVID-19 infection and promising therapeutic approaches**...As for common viral infections, the crucial event for the viral life cycle is the entry of genetic material inside the host cell, realized by the spike protein of the virus through its binding to host receptors and its activation by host proteases; this is followed by translation of the viral RNA into a polyprotein, exploiting the host cell machinery. The production of individual mature viral proteins is pivotal for replication and release of new virions. Several proteolytic enzymes either of the host and of the virus act in a concerted fashion to regulate and coordinate specific steps of the viral replication and assembly, such as (i) the entry of the virus, (ii) the maturation of the polyprotein and (iii) the assembly of the secreted virions for further diffusion. Therefore, proteases involved in these three steps are important targets, envisaging that molecules which interfere with their activity are promising therapeutic compounds. In this review, we will survey what is known up to now on the role of specific proteolytic enzymes in these three steps and of most promising compounds designed to impair this vicious cycle.

https://www.ncbi.nlm.nih.gov/pmc/articles/PMC7501082/


**A Randomized Controlled Trial of the Efficacy of Systemic Enzymes and Probiotics in the Resolution of Post-COVID Fatigue**...Muscle fatigue and cognitive disturbances persist in patients after recovery from acute COVID-19 disease. However, there are no specific treatments for post-COVID fatigue. Objective: To evaluate the efficacy and safety of the health supplements ImmunoSEB (systemic enzyme complex) and ProbioSEB CSC3 (probiotic complex) in patients suffering from COVID-19 induced fatigue. A randomized, multicentric, double blind, placebo-controlled trial was conducted in 200 patients with a complaint of post-COVID fatigue. The test arm (n = 100) received the oral supplements for 14 days and the control arm (n = 100) received a placebo. Treatment efficacy was compared using the Chalder Fatigue scale (CFQ-11), at various time points from days 1 to 14. The supplemental treatment resulted in resolution of fatigue in a greater percentage of subjects in the test vs. the control arm (91% vs. 15%) on day 14. Subjects in the test arm showed a significantly greater reduction in total as well as physical and mental fatigue scores at all time points vs. the control arm. The supplements were well tolerated with no adverse events reported. This study demonstrates that a 14 days supplementation of ImmunoSEB + ProbioSEB CSC3 resolves post-COVID-19 fatigue and can improve patients' functional status and quality of life.

https://www.ncbi.nlm.nih.gov/pmc/articles/PMC8472462/

**The enzymes in COVID-19: A review**...As enzymes are indispensable to uncountable biochemical reactions in the human body, it is not surprising that some enzymes are of relevance to COVID-19 pathophysiology. Past evidence from SARS-CoV and MERS-CoV outbreaks provided hints about the role of enzymes in SARS-CoV-2 infection. In this setting, ACE-2 is an enzyme of great importance since it is the cell entry receptor for SARS-CoV-2. Clinical data elucidate patterns of enzymatic alterations in COVID-19, which could be associated with organ damage, prognosis, and clinical complications. Further, viral mutations can create new disease behaviors, and these effects are related to the activity of enzymes. This review will discuss the main enzymes related to COVID-19, summarizing the findings on their role in viral entry mechanism, the consequences of their dysregulation, and the effects of SARS-CoV-2 mutations on them.

https://www.ncbi.nlm.nih.gov/pmc/articles/PMC8789385/

*"Enzyme production is often disturbed by COVID-19 infection."*

**Steven Magee**

# Digestive System

**COVID-19 and the Digestive System**...Although COVID-19 is principally defined by its respiratory symptoms, it is now clear that the virus can also affect the digestive system. In this review, we elaborate on the close relationship between COVID-19 and the digestive system, focusing on both the clinical findings and potential underlying mechanisms of COVID-19 gastrointestinal pathogenesis.

https://www.ncbi.nlm.nih.gov/pmc/articles/PMC7273952/

**COVID-19 and the digestive system: A comprehensive review**...Previous studies have indicated that SARS-CoV-2 ribonucleic acid could be detected in the feces of patients even after smear-negative respiratory samples. However, demonstration of confirmed fecal-oral transmission has been difficult. Clinical studies have shown an incidence rate of gastrointestinal (GI) symptoms ranging from 2% to 79.1% in patients with COVID-19. They may precede or accompany respiratory symptoms. The most common GI symptoms included nausea, diarrhea, and abdominal pain. In addition, some patients also had liver injury, pancreatic damage, and even acute mesenteric ischemia/thrombosis. Although the incidence rates reported in different centers were quite different, the digestive system was the clinical component of the COVID-19 section. Studies have shown that angiotensin-converting enzyme 2, the receptor of SARS-CoV-2, was not only expressed in the lungs, but also in the upper esophagus, small intestine, liver, and colon. The possible mechanism of GI symptoms in COVID-19 patients may include direct viral invasion into target cells, dysregulation of angiotensin-converting enzyme 2, immune-mediated tissue injury, and gut dysbiosis caused by microbiota. Additionally, numerous experiences, guidelines, recommendations, and position statements were published or released by different organizations and societies worldwide to optimize the management practice of outpatients, inpatients, and endoscopy in the era of COVID-19. In this review, based on our previous work and relevant literature, we mainly discuss potential fecal-oral transmission, GI manifestations, abdominal imaging findings, relevant pathophysiological mechanisms, and infection control and prevention measures in the time of COVID-19.

https://www.ncbi.nlm.nih.gov/pmc/articles/PMC8180220/

**Impact of COVID-19 on the Gastrointestinal Tract: A Clinical Review**...The gastrointestinal (GI) tract is known to have high expression of angiotensin-converting enzyme 2 (ACE2) receptors in the human body, making it prone to direct damage from the cellular invasion of severe acute respiratory syndrome coronavirus 2 (SARS-CoV-2). Numerous GI symptoms have been reported among patients with COVID-19. This systemic review details the mechanism and effects of COVID-19 on the GI tract along with the hepatobiliary and pancreatic systems.

https://www.ncbi.nlm.nih.gov/pmc/articles/PMC9017282/

**Digestive involvement in the Long-COVID syndrome**…The SARS-CoV-2 infection which caused a worldwide epidemic was considered first a lung disease. Later on, it was found that the disease caused by this virus, SARS-CoV-2, can affect most organs, including the digestive system. The long-term effects of this infection are now progressively detected and called Long-COVID. This review aims is to present the updated knowledge of the digestive sequelae after SARS-CoV-2 infection...The main symptoms that can occur in the long term are: diarrhea, nausea, vomiting, abdominal pain, along with increased liver enzymes. Patients with chronic diseases have a higher risk of developing long-term sequelae, but it is not documented that digestive sequelae are influenced by the presence of chronic diseases.

https://www.ncbi.nlm.nih.gov/pmc/articles/PMC9177081/

*"Gastrointestinal issues were commonly reported during COVID-19 infections."*

**Steven Magee**

## Kidneys

**COVID-19 and the kidney: time to take a closer look**...Although coronavirus disease (COVID-19) is primarily a respiratory disease, the kidney may be among the target organs of infection with severe acute respiratory syndrome coronavirus 2 (SARS-COV-2). Independently of baseline kidney function, acute kidney injury (AKI) is a common complication of COVID-19, associated with increased mortality and morbidity. Most frequently, COVID-19 causes acute tubular necrosis; however, in some cases, collapsing focal segmental glomerulosclerosis and direct viral tropism of the kidneys have also been documented. AKI secondary to COVID-19 has a multi-factorial origin. Even mild impairment of renal function is an independent risk factor for COVID-19 infection, hospitalisation and mortality. Dialysis patients also carry an increased risk of other severe COVID-related complications, including arrhythmias, shock, acute respiratory distress syndrome and acute heart failure. In such patients, COVID-19 may even present with atypical clinical symptoms, including gastrointestinal disorders and deterioration of mental status. More research is needed on the exact effects of SARS-CoV-2 on the kidneys. Finally, it remains to be proven whether the outcome of patients with kidney disease may be improved with anticipated vaccination programmes.

https://www.ncbi.nlm.nih.gov/pmc/articles/PMC8358250/

**COVID–19 and chronic kidney disease: an updated overview of reviews**...While COVID–19 mostly affects the lungs, different comorbidities can have an impact on its outcomes. We performed an overview of reviews to assess the effect of Chronic Kidney Disease (CKD) on contracting COVID–19, hospitalization, mortality, and disease severity...an increased risk of hospitalization in patients with CKD and COVID–19...Evidence consistently demonstrated an increased risk of mortality and hospitalization in patients with CKD and COVID–19.

https://www.ncbi.nlm.nih.gov/pmc/articles/PMC8747880/


**Mechanisms of COVID-19-induced kidney injury and current pharmacotherapies**...While significant evidence is currently available online and targets various aspects of the disease, both inflammatory and noninflammatory kidney manifestations secondary to COVID-19 infection are still largely underrepresented. In this review, we summarized current knowledge about COVID-19-related kidney manifestations, their pathologic mechanisms as well as various pharmacotherapies used to treat patients with COVID-19. We also shed light on the effect of these medications on kidney functions that can further enhance renal damage secondary to the illness...renal manifestations are often seen in COVID-19 patients, and they are associated with increased mortality in subjects admitted to the ICU. It is becoming clear that SARS-CoV-2 particles strike the kidneys in addition to the cytokine storm that perpetuates renal damage in these patients. In the same view, it is evident that some of the currently approved medications to treat COVID-19 patients influenced renal function and must be administered with extreme care. Nonetheless, while some of the adopted vaccines were associated with minimal change disease, none of them was discontinued. Thus, kidney safety in COVID-19 patients remains of utmost concern view the central role that kidneys play in regulating blood pressure and filtering blood from toxic substances. Therefore, constant monitoring of kidneys' fitness along with cardiac hemodynamics in COVID-19 subjects is imperative to reduce the burden of COVID-19 on human lives. This involves close cardiorenal monitoring to prevent kidney damage in COVID-19 patients.

https://www.ncbi.nlm.nih.gov/pmc/articles/PMC8606168/


**Kidney Outcomes in Long COVID**...Patients who survive coronavirus disease 2019 (COVID-19) are at higher risk of post-acute sequelae involving pulmonary and several extrapulmonary organ systems—generally referred to as long COVID. However, a detailed assessment of kidney outcomes in long COVID is not yet available. Here we show that, beyond the acute phase of illness, 30-day survivors of COVID-19 exhibited higher risks of AKI, eGFR decline, ESKD, major adverse kidney events (MAKE), and steeper longitudinal decline in eGFR. The risks of kidney outcomes increased according to the severity of the acute infection (categorized by care setting into non-hospitalized, hospitalized, and admitted to intensive care). The findings provide insight into the long-term consequences of COVID-19 on kidney outcomes and suggest that post-acute COVID-19 care should include attention to kidney function and disease...The implications of our findings are clear. Given the large number of people infected with COVID-19 (>43 million people in the United States, and >234 million globally), and given that estimates by the World Health Organization suggest that around 10% of people infected with COVID-19 may experience post-acute sequelae, the numbers of people with long COVID-19 in need of post–COVID-19 care will likely be staggering and will present substantial strain on already overwhelmed health systems. Governments and health systems around the world are establishing post-acute COVID-19 clinics to attend to the needs of people with postacute COVID-19 sequelae. The optimal composition of those clinics is not yet clear. The higher risks of adverse kidney outcomes reported in this study highlights the need for integration of kidney care as a component of the multidisciplinary post-acute COVID-19 care. Our estimates of the burden of kidney sequelae may also be useful to inform capacity planning.

https://www.ncbi.nlm.nih.gov/pmc/articles/PMC8806085/


*"The kidneys are vulnerable to hypoxic damage."*

**Steven Magee**

## Liver

**COVID-19 and the liver: What do we know so far?**...The initial uncertainty and fear of cross transmission of severe acute respiratory syndrome coronavirus 2 (SARS-CoV-2) have changed the routine management of patients with pre-existing liver diseases, hepatocellular carcinoma, and patients either listed for or received a liver transplant. COVID-19 is best described as a multisystem disease caused by SARS-CoV-2, and it can cause acute liver injury or decompensation of the pre-existing liver disease. There has been considerable research on the pathophysiology, infection transmission, and treatment of COVID-19 in the last few months. The pathogenesis of liver involvement in COVID-19 includes viral cytotoxicity, the secondary effect of immune dysregulation, hypoxia resulting from respiratory failure, ischemic damage caused by vascular endotheliitis, congestion because of right heart failure, or drug-induced liver injury. Patients with chronic liver diseases, cirrhosis, and hepatocellular carcinoma are at high risk for severe COVID-19 and mortality. The phase III trials of recently approved vaccines for SARS-CoV-2 did not include enough patients with pre-existing liver diseases and excluded immunocompromised patients or those on immunomodulators. This article reviews the currently published research on the effect of COVID-19 on the liver and the management of patients with pre-existing liver disease, including SARS-CoV-2 vaccines...Emerging research suggests that liver injury is common in COVID-19 patients and associated with worse outcomes. Patients with CLD and post liver transplant patients are at risk of SARS-CoV-2 infection, with an increased risk of complications and mortality. The management of this vulnerable group of patients should be prioritized based on their clinical condition, strategies to reduce cross transmission, and optimizing limited resources. Liver transplant and HCC management programs should be modified depending on the prevalence of community transmission of SARS-CoV-2. Specific management issues should be considered during the treatment of COVID-19 in patients with pre-existing liver diseases.

https://www.ncbi.nlm.nih.gov/pmc/articles/PMC8173343/

**Involvement of the Liver in COVID-19: A Systematic Review**...In this review, we have outlined the important liver manifestations of COVID-19 and discussed the possible underlying pathophysiological mechanisms and their diagnosis and management. Factors that may contribute to hepatic involvement in COVID-19 include direct viral cytopathic effects, exaggerated immune responses/systemic inflammatory response syndrome, hypoxia-induced changes, vascular changes due to coagulopathy, endothelitis, cardiac congestion from right heart failure, and drug-induced liver injury. The majority of COVID-19-associated liver symptoms are mild and self-limiting. Thus management is generally supportive. Liver function tests and abdominal imaging are the primary investigations done in relation to liver involvement in COVID-19 patients. However, imaging findings are nonspecific. Severe acute respiratory syndrome coronavirus 2 RNA has been found in liver biopsies. However, there is limited place for liver biopsy in the clinical context, as it does not influence management. Although, the management is supportive in the majority of patients without previous liver disease, special emphasis is needed in those with nonalcoholic fatty liver disease, cirrhosis, hepatocellular carcinoma, hepatitis B and C infections, and alcoholic liver disease, and in liver transplant recipients.

https://www.ncbi.nlm.nih.gov/pmc/articles/PMC8991364/

**Patterns of liver profile disturbance in patients with COVID-19**...Fever and cough are the most common clinical symptoms of coronavirus disease 2019 (COVID-19), but complications (such as pneumonia, respiratory distress syndrome, and multiorgan failure) can occur in people with additional comorbidities. COVID-19 may be a new cause of liver disease, as liver profile disturbance is one of the most common findings among patients. The molecular mechanism underlying this phenomenon, however, is still unknown. In this paper, we review the most current research on the patterns of change in liver profile among patients with COVID-19, the possible explanation for these findings, and the relation to pre-existing liver disease in these patients...COVID-19-related liver injury is usually mild and of a hepatocellular pattern. It may affect a significant proportion of patients, especially those with a more severe disease course.

https://www.ncbi.nlm.nih.gov/pmc/articles/PMC8895188/

**Long COVID-19 Liver Manifestation in Children**...OBJECTIVES: Severe acute respiratory syndrome coronavirus 2, the novel coronavirus responsible for coronavirus disease (COVID-19), has been a major cause of morbidity and mortality worldwide. Gastrointestinal and hepatic manifestations during acute disease have been reported extensively in the literature. Post-COVID-19 cholangiopathy has been increasingly reported in adults. In children, data are sparse. Our aim was to describe pediatric patients who recovered from COVID-19 and later presented with liver injury. METHODS: This is a retrospective case series study of pediatric patients with post-COVID-19 liver manifestations. We collected data on demographics, medical history, clinical presentation, laboratory results, imaging, histology, treatment, and outcome. RESULTS: We report 5 pediatric patients who recovered from COVID-19 and later presented with liver injury. Two types of clinical presentation were distinguishable. Two infants aged 3 and 5 months, previously healthy, presented with acute liver failure that rapidly progressed to liver transplantation. Their liver explant showed massive necrosis with cholangiolar proliferation and lymphocytic infiltrate. Three children, 2 aged 8 years and 1 aged 13 years, presented with hepatitis with cholestasis. Two children had a liver biopsy significant for lymphocytic portal and parenchyma inflammation, along with bile duct proliferations. All 3 were started on steroid treatment; liver enzymes improved, and they were weaned successfully from treatment. For all 5 patients, extensive etiology workup for infectious and metabolic etiologies was negative. CONCLUSIONS: We report 2 distinct patterns of potentially long

COVID-19 liver manifestations in children with common clinical, radiological, and histopathological characteristics after a thorough workup excluded other known etiologies.

https://www.ncbi.nlm.nih.gov/research/coronavirus/publication/35687535

*"Liver damage was a common outcome of COVID-19 infections."*

**Steven Magee**

## Monster Energy Drink

Green "Monster Energy" drink contains the following:

- Riboflavin (B2) 260%.

- Niacin (B3) 250%.

- Vitamin B6 240%.

- Vitamin B12 500%.

- Glucose.

- Taurine.

- Panax ginger extract.

- L-Carnitine.

- Caffeine.

- Glucuronolactone.

- Inositol.

- Gurana extract.

- Maltodextrin.

**The serum amino acid profile in COVID-19**...Amino acid metabolism, in particular, contains significant clues in terms of the development and prevention of many diseases. Therefore, this study aimed to compare amino acid profile of COVID 19 and healthy subject. In this study, the amino acid profiles of patients with asymptomatic, mild, moderate, and severe/critical SARS-CoV-2 infection were scanned with LC–MS/MS. The amino acid profile encompassing 30 amino acids in 142 people including 30 control and 112 COVID-19 patients was examined. 20 amino acids showed significant differences when compared to the control group in COVID-19 patient groups with different levels of severity in the statistical analyses conducted. It was detected that the branched-chain amino acids (BCAAs) changed in correlation with one another, and l-2-aminobutyric acid and l-phenylalanine had biomarker potential for COVID-19. Moreover, it was concluded that l-2-aminobutyric acid could provide prognostic information about the course of the disease. We believe that a new viewpoint will develop regarding the diagnosis, treatment, and prognosis as a result of the evaluation of the serum amino acid profiles of COVID-19 patients. Determining l-phenylalanine and l-2-aminobutyric levels can be used in laboratories as a COVID-19-biomarker. Also, supplementing COVID patients with taurine and BCAAs can be beneficial for treatment protocols.

https://www.ncbi.nlm.nih.gov/pmc/articles/PMC8487804/

**The role of taurine derivatives in the putative therapy of COVID-19-induced inflammation**...With the world's current focus being on developing definite therapeutics, the issue of cytokine storm plaguing COVID-19 infection needs to be addressed. The proinflammatory process contributing to cytokine storm substantiates the need for targeted immune-suppressive treatment. The efficacy of taurine derivatives as an infection barrier is well documented in literature, and we believe its putative anti-inflammatory role should be regarded as a promising available therapeutic approach in COVID-19 patient management, for which minimal to no side effects are known.

https://www.ncbi.nlm.nih.gov/pmc/articles/PMC7889472/

**Therapeutic potential of ginger against COVID-19: Is there enough evidence?**...In addition to the respiratory system, severe acute respiratory syndrome coronavirus 2 (SARS-CoV-2) strikes other systems, including the digestive, circulatory, urogenital, and even the central nervous system, as its receptor angiotensin-converting enzyme 2 (ACE2) is expressed in various organs, such as lungs, intestine, heart, esophagus, kidneys, bladder, testis, liver, and brain. Different mechanisms, in particular, massive virus replication, extensive apoptosis and necrosis of the lung-related epithelial and endothelial cells, vascular leakage, hyper-inflammatory responses, overproduction of pro-inflammatory mediators, cytokine storm, oxidative stress, downregulation of ACE2, and impairment of the renin-angiotensin system contribute to the COVID-19 pathogenesis. Currently, COVID-19 is a global pandemic with no specific anti-viral treatment. The favorable capabilities of the ginger were indicated in patients suffering from osteoarthritis, neurodegenerative disorders, rheumatoid arthritis, type 2 diabetes, respiratory distress, liver diseases and primary dysmenorrheal. Ginger or its compounds exhibited strong anti-inflammatory and anti-oxidative influences in numerous animal models. This review provides evidence regarding the potential effects of ginger against SARS-CoV-2 infection and highlights its antiviral, anti-inflammatory, antioxidative, and immunomodulatory impacts in an attempt to consider this plant as an alternative therapeutic agent for COVID-19 treatment.

https://www.ncbi.nlm.nih.gov/pmc/articles/PMC8492833/

**Ginger supplement significantly reduced length of hospital stay in individuals with COVID-19**...Among all participants, a significant reduction in hospitalization time (the difference between the treatment and control groups was 2.4 d, 95% CI 1.6–3.2) was detected in response to the ginger supplement. This effect was more pronounced in men, participants aged 60 years or older, and participants with pre-existing medical conditions, relative to their counterparts (P-interactions < 0.05 for all)...Ginger supplement significantly shortened the length of stay of hospitalized individuals with COVID-19.

https://www.ncbi.nlm.nih.gov/pmc/articles/PMC9795954/

**Inositol and vitamin D may naturally protect human reproduction and women undergoing assisted reproduction from Covid-19 risk**...Pregnant women represent a risk category for increased abortion rates and vertical transmission with adverse events on the newborns has been recently confirmed. The scientific world is struggling for finding an effective cure for counteracting symptomatology. Today, there are many therapeutic proposes but none of them can effectively counteract the infection. Moreover, many of these compounds show important side effects not justifying their use. Scientific literature reports an immune system over-reaction through interleukins-6 activation. In this regard, the possibility to control the immune system represents a possible strategy for counteracting the onset of COVID-19 symptomatology. Vitamin D deficiency shows increased susceptibility to acute viral respiratory infections. Moreover, Vitamin D seems involved in host protection from different virus species by modulating activation and release of cytokines. Myo-inositol down-regulates the expression of IL-6 by phosphatidyl-inositol-3-kinase (PI3K) pathway. Furthermore, myo-inositol is the precursor of phospholipids in the surfactant and it is applied for inducing surfactant synthesis in infants for treating respiratory distress syndrome (RDS). This review aims to summarize the evidence about COVID-19 infection in pregnant women and to encourage the scientific community to investigate the use of Vitamin D and Myo-inositol which could represent a possible preventive treatment for pregnant women or women undergoing assisted reproductive technologies (ART).

https://www.ncbi.nlm.nih.gov/pmc/articles/PMC7833496/

**Inositol and pulmonary function. Could myo-inositol treatment downregulate inflammation and cytokine release syndrome in SARS-CoV-2?**...Preliminary data point out that dramatic increase in IL-6 and subsequent cytokine release syndrome may account for the development of fatal interstitial pneumonia. Inhibition of IL-6 by blocking its specific receptor with monoclonal antibodies has been advocated as a promising attempt. Here we assess the potential utility of myo-Inositol, a polyol already in use for treating the newborn Respiratory Distress Syndrome, in downregulating the inflammatory response upon Sars-CoV-2 infection. Myo-Inositol proved to reduce IL-6 levels in a number of conditions and to mitigate the inflammatory cascade, while being devoid of any significant side effects. It is tempting to speculate that inositol could be beneficial in managing the most dreadful effects of Sars-CoV-2 infection.

https://pubmed.ncbi.nlm.nih.gov/32271462/

**Role of inositol to improve surfactant functions and reduce IL-6 levels: A potential adjuvant strategy for SARS-CoV-2 pneumonia?**…Although the infection can be asymptomatic, several cases develop severe pneumonia and acute respiratory distress syndrome (ARDS) characterized by high levels of pro-inflammatory cytokines, primarily interleukin (IL)-6. Based on available data, the severity of ARDS and serum levels of IL-6 are key determinants for the prognosis.  In this scenario, available in vitro and in vivo data suggested that myo-inositol is able to increase the synthesis and function of the surfactant phosphatidylinositol, acting on the phosphoinositide 3-kinase (PI3K)-regulated signaling, with amelioration of both immune system and oxygenation at the bronchoalveolar level. In addition, myo-inositol has been found able to decrease the levels of IL-6 in several experimental settings, due to an effect on the inositol-requiring enzyme 1 (IRE1)-X-box-binding protein 1 (XBP1) and on the signal transducer and activator of transcription 3 (STAT3) pathways. In this scenario, treatment with myo-inositol may be able to reduce IL-6 dependent inflammatory response and improve oxygenation in patients with severe ARDS by SARS-CoV-2. In addition, the action of myo-inositol on IRE1 endonuclease activity may also inhibit the replication of SARS-CoV-2, as was reported for the respiratory syncytial virus. Since the available data are extremely limited, if this potential therapeutic approach will be considered valid in the clinical practice, the necessary future investigations should aim to identify the best dose, administration route (oral, intravenous and/or aerosol nebulization), and cluster(s) of patients which may get beneficial effects from this treatment.

https://www.ncbi.nlm.nih.gov/pmc/articles/PMC7480225/


**Medicinal Herbs in the Relief of Neurological, Cardiovascular, and Respiratory Symptoms after COVID-19 Infection A Literature Review**...COVID-19 infection causes complications, even in people who have had a mild course of the disease. The most dangerous seem to be neurological ailments: anxiety, depression, mixed anxiety–depressive (MAD) syndromes, and irreversible dementia. These conditions can negatively affect the respiratory system, circulatory system, and heart functioning. We believe that phytotherapy can be helpful in all of these conditions. Clinical trials confirm this possibility. The work presents plant materials (Valeriana officinalis, Melissa officinalis, Passiflora incarnata, Piper methysticum, Humulus lupulus, Ballota nigra, Hypericum perforatum, Rhodiola rosea, Lavandula officinalis, Paullinia cupana, Ginkgo biloba, Murraya koenigii, Crataegus monogyna and oxyacantha, Hedera helix, Polygala senega, Pelargonium sidoides, Lichen islandicus, Plantago lanceolata) and their dominant compounds (valeranon, valtrate, apigenin, citronellal, isovitexin, isoorientin, methysticin, humulone, farnesene, acteoside, hypericin, hyperforin, biapigenin, rosavidin, salidroside, linalool acetate, linalool, caffeine, ginkgolide, bilobalide, mihanimbine, epicatechin, hederacoside C,α-hederine, presegenin, umckalin, 6,7,8-trixydroxybenzopyranone disulfate, fumaroprotocetric acid, protolichesteric acid, aucubin, acteoside) responsible for their activity. It also shows the possibility of reducing post-COVID-19 neurological, respiratory, and cardiovascular complications, which can affect the functioning of the nervous system.

https://www.ncbi.nlm.nih.gov/pmc/articles/PMC9220793/


**Amazonian fruits with potential effects on COVID-19 by inflammaging modulation: A narrative review**...The COVID-19 pandemic had a great impact on the mortality of older adults and, chronic non- transmissible diseases (CNTDs) patients, likely previous inflammaging condition that is common in these subjects. It is possible that functional foods could attenuate viral infection conditions such as SARS-CoV-2 (severe acute respiratory syndrome coronavirus 2), the causal agent of COVID-19 pandemic. Previous evidence suggested that some fruits consumed by Amazonian Diet from Pre-Colombian times could present relevant proprieties to decrease of COVID-19 complications such as oxidative-cytokine storm. In this narrative review we identified five potential Amazonian fruits: açai berry (Euterpe oleracea), camu-camu (Myrciaria dubia), cocoa (Theobroma cacao), Brazil nuts (Bertholletia excelsa), and guaraná (Paullinia cupana). Data showed that these Amazonian fruits present antioxidant, anti-inflammatory and other immunomodulatory activities that could attenuate the impact of inflammaging states that potentially decrease the evolution of COVID-19 complications. The evidence compiled here supports the complementary experimental and clinical studies exploring these fruits as nutritional supplement during COVID-19 infection. PRACTICAL APPLICATIONS: These fruits, in their natural form, are often limited to their region, or exported to other places in the form of frozen pulp or powder. But there are already some companies producing food supplements in the form of capsules, in the form of oils and even functional foods enriched with these fruits. This practice is common in Brazil and tends to expand to the international market.

https://pubmed.ncbi.nlm.nih.gov/36240164/


**"Energy drinks may have an application in treating COVID-19."**

**Steven Magee**

## Coffee

**Possible Beneficial Actions of Caffeine in SARS-CoV-2**...The consumption of caffeine has been suggested primarily because it improves exercise performance, reduces fatigue, and increases wakefulness and awareness. Caffeine has been proven to be an effective anti-inflammatory and immunomodulator. In airway smooth muscle, it has bronchodilator effects mainly due to its activity as a phosphodiesterase inhibitor and adenosine receptor antagonist. In addition, a recent published document has suggested the potential antiviral activity of this drug using in silico molecular dynamics and molecular docking; in this regard, caffeine might block the viral entrance into host cells by inhibiting the formation of a receptor-binding domain and the angiotensin-converting enzyme complex and, additionally, might reduce viral replication by the inhibition of the activity of 3-chymotrypsin-like proteases. Here, we discuss how caffeine through certain mechanisms of action could be beneficial in SARS-CoV-2. Nevertheless, further studies are required for validation through in vitro and in vivo models.

https://www.ncbi.nlm.nih.gov/pmc/articles/PMC8196824/

**Caffeine and caffeine-containing pharmaceuticals as promising inhibitors for 3-chymotrypsin-like protease of SARS-CoV-2**...This study investigates the inhibitory effect of SARS-CoV-2 3-chymotrypsin-like protease (3CLpro) using caffeine and caffeine-containing pharmaceuticals (3CPs) based on molecular dynamics simulations and free energy calculations by means of molecular mechanics-Poisson–Boltzmann surface area (MMPBSA) and molecular mechanics-generalized-Born surface area (MMGBSA). Of these 3CPs, seven drugs approved by the US-Food and Drug Administration have shown a good binding affinity to the catalytic residues of 3CLpro of His41 and Cys145: caffeine, theophylline, dyphylline, pentoxifylline, linagliptin, bromotheophylline and istradefylline. Their binding affinity score ranged from –4.9 to –8.6 kcal/mol. The molecular dynamic simulation in an aqueous solution of docked complexes demonstrated that the 3CPs conformations bound to the active sites of 3CLpro during 200 ns molecular dynamics simulations. The free energy of binding also confirms the stability of the 3CPs–3CLpro complexes. To our knowledge, this in silico study shows for the first time very inexpensive drugs available in large quantities that can be potential inhibitors against 3CLpro. In particular, the repurposing of linagliptin, and caffeine are recommended for COVID-19 treatment after in vitro, in vivo and clinical trial validation.

https://www.ncbi.nlm.nih.gov/pmc/articles/PMC7594182/


**Disorders of the Cholinergic System in COVID-19 Era-A Review of the Latest Research**...research has been conducted on the changes that SARS-CoV-2 may cause in the cholinergic system. The aim of this study is to review the latest research from the years 2020/2021 regarding disorders in the cholinergic system caused by the SARS-CoV-2 virus. As a result of the research, it was found that the presence of the COVID-19 virus disrupts the activity of the cholinergic system, for example, causing the development of myasthenia gravis or a change in acetylcholine activity. The SARS-CoV-2 spike protein has a sequence similar to neurotoxins, capable of binding nicotinic acetylcholine receptors (nAChR). This may be proof that SARS-CoV-2 can bind nAChR. Nicotine and caffeine have similar structures to antiviral drugs, capable of binding angiotensin-converting enzyme 2 (ACE 2) epitopes that are recognized by SARS-CoV-2, with the potential to inhibit the formation of the ACE 2/SARS-CoV-2 complex. The blocking is enhanced when nicotine and caffeine are used together with antiviral drugs. This is proof that nAChR agonists can be used along with antiviral drugs in COVID-19 therapy. As a result, it is possible to develop COVID-19 therapies that use these compounds to reduce cytokine production. Another promising therapy is non-invasive stimulation of the vagus nerve, which soothes the body's cytokine storm. Research on the influence of COVID-19 on the cholinergic system is an area that should continue to be developed as there is a need for further research. It can be firmly stated that COVID-19 causes a dysregulation of the cholinergic system, which leads to a need for further research, because there are many promising therapies that will prevent the SARS-CoV-2 virus from binding to the nicotinic receptor. There is a need for further research, both in vitro and in vivo. It should be noted that in the functioning of the cholinergic system and its connection with the activity of the COVID-19 virus, there might be many promising dependencies and solutions.

https://pubmed.ncbi.nlm.nih.gov/35054856/

**Why Methodology Is Important: Coffee as a Candidate Treatment for COVID-19?**...Patients receiving the TMX treatment had a significantly shorter hospital stay (9.5 vs. 15 days, p < 0.05). Moreover, TMX decreased the use of antibiotics and the extension of pulmonary lesions in the CT-scans. These results lead to the conclusion that the 1,3,7-Trimethylxanthine (TMX), the active molecule of the patients' morning coffee beverage, is a potential treatment for COVID-19 infection.

https://www.ncbi.nlm.nih.gov/pmc/articles/PMC7698499/

**Prevention and Management of Type 2 Diabetes and Metabolic Syndrome in the Time of COVID-19: Should We Add a Cup of Coffee?**...Recent evidence shows that COVID-19 patients with existing metabolic disorders, such as diabetes and metabolic syndrome, are exposed to a high risk of morbidity and mortality. At the same time, in order to manage the pandemic, the health authorities around the world are advising people to stay at home. This results in decreased physical activity and an increased consumption of an unhealthy diet, which often leads to an increase in body weight, risk for diabetes, insulin resistance, and metabolic syndrome, and thus, paradoxically, to a high risk of morbidity and mortality due to COVID-19 complications. Here we summarize the evidence demonstrating that the promotion of a healthy life style, including physical activity and a dietary intake of natural polyphenols present in coffee and tea, has the potential to improve the prevention and management of insulin resistance and diabetes in the time of COVID-19 pandemic. Particularly, it would be pertinent to evaluate further the potential positive effects of coffee beverages, rich in natural polyphenols, as an adjuvant therapy for COVID-19, which appear not to be studied sufficiently.

https://pubmed.ncbi.nlm.nih.gov/33123550/

*"Coffee may be a natural treatment for COVID-19."*

**Steven Magee**

## Hydration

**Hypotheses about sub-optimal hydration in the weeks before coronavirus disease (COVID-19) as a risk factor for dying from COVID-19...**To address urgent need for strategies to limit mortality from coronavirus disease 2019 (COVID-19), this review describes experimental, clinical and epidemiological evidence that suggests that chronic sub-optimal hydration in the weeks before infection might increase risk of COVID-19 mortality in multiple ways. Sub-optimal hydration is associated with key risk factors for COVID-19 mortality, including older age, male sex, race-ethnicity and chronic disease. Chronic hypertonicity, total body water deficit and/or hypovolemia cause multiple intracellular and/or physiologic adaptations that preferentially retain body water and favor positive total body water balance when challenged by infection. Via effects on serum/glucocorticoid-regulated kinase 1 (SGK1) signaling, aldosterone, tumor necrosis factor-alpha (TNF-alpha), vascular endothelial growth factor (VEGF), aquaporin 5 (AQP5) and/or Na+/K+-ATPase, chronic sub-optimal hydration in the weeks before exposure to COVID-19 may conceivably result in: greater abundance of angiotensin converting enzyme 2 (ACE2) receptors in the lung, which increases likelihood of COVID-19 infection, lung epithelial cells which are pre-set for exaggerated immune response, increased capacity for capillary leakage of fluid into the airway space, and/or reduced capacity for both passive and active transport of fluid out of the airways. The hypothesized hydration effects suggest hypotheses regarding strategies for COVID-19 risk reduction, such as public health recommendations to increase intake of drinking water, hydration screening alongside COVID-19 testing, and treatment tailored to the pre-infection hydration condition. Hydration may link risk factors and pathways in a unified mechanism for COVID-19 mortality. Attention to hydration holds potential to reduce COVID-19 mortality and disparities via at least 5 pathways simultaneously.

https://www.ncbi.nlm.nih.gov/pmc/articles/PMC7467030/

**Hyponatremia due to excessive water intake in COVID-19 patients: case series study**...Literatures revealed syndrome of inappropriate antidiuretic hormone (SIADH) as the most common mechanism of hyponatremia in COVID-19. However, it is important to rule out other etiologies of hyponatremia...History revealed that the patients were drinking large amounts of water, around 4–5 L/day, due of certain reasons: one patient had dysgeusia, and the other three patients thought that excessive drinking of water is beneficial for COVID-19 infection...Fluid restriction up to 1.5 L/day showed dramatic improvement of their sodium blood level. The patients are discharged in a stable condition…In COVID-19 patients, hyponatremia not only is secondary to SIADH but can also be due to other etiologies. Hyponatremia can be induced by excessive water drinking and considered an extremely rare reported cases.

https://www.ncbi.nlm.nih.gov/pmc/articles/PMC9510225/

**Fluid and Electrolyte Disturbances in COVID-19 and Their Complications**...The virus infects the host by binding to the angiotensin-converting enzyme 2 (ACE2) receptors. Due to the presence of ACE2 receptors in the kidneys and gastrointestinal (GI) tract, kidneys and GI tract damage arising from the virus can be seen in patients and can cause acute conditions such as acute kidney injury (AKI) and digestive problems for the patient. One of the complications of kidneys and GI involvement in COVID-19 is fluid and electrolyte disturbances. The most common ones of these disorders are hyponatremia, hypernatremia, hypokalemia, hypocalcemia, hypochloremia, hypervolemia, and hypovolemia, which if left untreated, cause many problems for patients and even increase mortality. Fluid and electrolyte disturbances are more common in hospitalized and intensive care patients. Children are also at greater risk for fluid and electrolyte disturbances complications. Therefore, clinicians should pay special attention to the fluid and electrolyte status of patients. Changes in fluid and electrolyte levels can be a good indicator of disease progression.

https://www.ncbi.nlm.nih.gov/pmc/articles/PMC8060100/

**COVID-19 symptoms are reduced by targeted hydration of the nose, larynx and trachea**...Dehydration of the upper airways increases risks of respiratory diseases from COVID-19 to asthma and COPD. We find in human volunteer studies involving 464 human subjects in Germany, the US, and India that respiratory droplet generation increases by up to 4 orders of magnitude in dehydration-associated states of advanced age (n = 357), elevated BMI-age (n = 148), strenuous exercise (n = 20) and SARS-CoV-2 infection (n = 87), and falls with hydration of the nose, larynx and trachea by calcium-rich hypertonic salts. We also find in a protocol of exercise-induced airway dehydration that hydration of the airways by calcium-rich salts increases oxygenation relative to a non-treatment control ($P < 0.05$) In a random control study of COVID-19 positive subjects (n = 40), thrice-a-day delivery of the calcium-rich hypertonic salts (active) suppressed respiratory droplet generation by 51% ± 11% and increased oxygen saturation over three days of treatment by 48.08% ± 9.61% ($P < 0.001$), while no changes were observed in the nasal-saline control group. Self-reported symptoms significantly declined in the active group and did not decline in the control group. Hydration of the upper airways appears promising as a non-drug approach for reducing risks of respiratory diseases such as COVID-19.

https://pubmed.ncbi.nlm.nih.gov/35351914/

**Oral hydration therapy is an alternative approach to prevent nausea and vomiting in patients with COVID-19: A letter to the editor**...COVID-19 leads to gastrointestinal symptoms such as nausea and vomiting. Dehydration can reduce the appetite of patients with COVID-19. Oral hydration therapy can prevent nausea and vomiting in patients with COVID-19.

https://www.ncbi.nlm.nih.gov/pmc/articles/PMC8815285/

**Dietary Recommendations for Post-COVID-19 Syndrome**...At the beginning of the coronavirus disease (COVID-19) pandemic, global efforts focused on containing the spread of the virus and avoiding contagion. Currently, it is evident that health professionals should deal with the overall health status of COVID-19 survivors. Indeed, novel findings have identified post-COVID-19 syndrome, which is characterized by malnutrition, loss of fat-free mass, and low-grade inflammation. In addition, the recovery might be complicated by persistent functional impairment (i.e., fatigue and muscle weakness, dysphagia, appetite loss, and taste/smell alterations) as well as psychological distress. Therefore, the appropriate evaluation of nutritional status (assessment of dietary intake, anthropometrics, and body composition) is one of the pillars in the management of these patients. On the other hand, personalized dietary recommendations represent the best strategy to ensure recovery. Therefore, this review aimed to collect available evidence on the role of nutrients and their supplementation in post-COVID-19 syndrome to provide a practical guideline to nutritionists to tailor dietary interventions for patients recovering from COVID-19 infections...adequate hydration (30 mL/kg actual body weight) is important for the complete recovery of patients with post-COVID-19 syndrome. Therefore, these patients should increase their daily fluid intake (2.5–3 L/day) by consuming water, milk, fruit juice, broth, sports drinks, coffee, and tea.

https://www.ncbi.nlm.nih.gov/pmc/articles/PMC8954128/


*"Optimal hydration is part of the treatment for COVID-19."*

**Steven Magee**

## <u>Altitude Hypersensitivity</u>

Coronavirus damages the lungs and many people have been diagnosed with small airways disease after developing long COVID.  Damaged lungs can develop pressure sensitivities.  This may bring on altitude and weather sensitivities.  A low or high pressure weather system passing through your area may make you sick!  Changing altitude by flying, driving, vacationing, hiking or skiing may make you sick.  Living at altitude may keep you in a permanent state of sickness from hypoxic altitude sickness health issues.  If you are on a CPAP or BiPAP machine, these may may you sickly from the pressurized air they feed to you!  If you have had coronavirus, you should be watching for these pressure related health issues!

When I discovered I had altitude hypersensitivity and I was developing altitude sickness at just 1,000 feet, my initial thought was it was probably a life long condition.  However, experiments with nutritional supplements in combination with regular altitude exposures were revealing the condition was reducing in severity.

I had a lucky break in this research and that came from my ex-girlfriend.  During the relationship, she had been complaining of a lack of sex drive and a lack of interest in sex.  She believed she was in menopause.  As such, I bought her a menopause support supplement called "Amberen" that was supposed to reduce the symptoms of menopause.  However, she refused to take it.

Wondering what to do with the Amberen I now owned, I looked up the formulation and found it had no female hormones in it.  It was just a nutritional support supplement.  I could see no reason why a man could not take it.  A daily dose of Amberen contains a 400 mg blend of the following:

- Ammonium Succinate.

- Calcium Disuccinate.

- Monosodium L-Glutamate.

- Glycine.

- Magnesium Disuccinate.

- Zinc Difumarate.

- Tocopheryl Acetate.


The manufacturer states: *"Amberen contains a proprietary blend of bioactive antioxidants, amino acids, minerals and vitamin E."*

So I started to take it in June 2022.  A week after taking the Amberen, I did an altitude test.  I took my body up from 600 feet above sea level to 4,024 feet and much to my surprise noticed no symptoms that could make a diagnosis of altitude hypersensitivity. A few days later I took my body from 140 feet above sea level to 6,632 feet and again saw no symptoms that could make a diagnosis of altitude hypersensitivity.

This was the first time this had occurred during altitude testing.  The Amberen had changed the body chemistry.  I had noticed nerve pains in my face accompanied by twitching since I had been taking this supplement, so something was changing in the body regarding the nervous system.

The Amberen had fixed things!  Why was this?  Because I was age 52, I was in "Manopause".  Manopause is the male equivalent of the female menopause.  Just like aged females, the hormones also change in men after forty years of age.  Hormone decline occurs in both sexes after age forty.  But was there any evidence it could be the Amberen?

I took a look at the Amberen website and found this statement: *"Glycine: An amino acid involved in the processes regulating brain-cell activity.  In combination with magnesium, it makes brain mitochondria more resistant to low-oxygen conditions (hypoxia), which, in turn, results in the normalization of the psycho-emotional balance in the body."*

https://amberen.com/am-ingredients

So one of the ingredients of Amberen is a known treatment for hypoxia!  I was right!  Increasing altitude causes hypoxia and glycine treats it.  To confirm the information was correct on the Amberen website, I did an internet search on "glycine altitude" and found numerous articles about its beneficial effects at altitude.

After one month of taking Amberen:

- Regular altitude testing from sea level up to 6,632 feet was showing no evidence of altitude hypersensitivity.

- The side effects were:
  - Nerve pains in my face.
  - Facial muscles twitching.
  - Insomnia.
  - Mild headaches.
  - Mild heart pains.
  - All side effects subsided after one month of Amberen administration.

Amberen treats altitude hypersensitivity.  Altitude hypersensitivity at 1,000 feet returned during minimum supplement testing and this indicated it was one of the removed supplements that was causing it.  Reviewing my notes indicated that it had followed the removal of Acetyl-L-Carnitine HCl.  Taking L-Carnitine L-Tartrate at 500mg daily cleared up the altitude hypersensitivity.

Why did I switch from Acetyl-L-Carnitine HCl to L-Carnitine L-Tartrate?  I could not purchase Acetyl-L-Carnitine HCl at the time, due to the COVID-19 pandemic shortages.  L-Carnitine L-Tartrate was the closest thing to it that was available for purchase.

The question arose of what was the minimum amount of supplements needed to prevent altitude hypersensitivity from occurring?  I removed all supplements with the exception of

Amberen and L-Carnitine L-Tartrate and continued to be free of altitude hypersensitivity.  I did see some adverse reactions to L-Carnitine L-Tartrate as I raised the dose to 500 mg 4 times daily (total 2,000 mg daily):

- Day 1: No symptoms.

- Day 2: Hungry all day long and overeating.

- Day 3: Fatigued all day long and stayed in bed.  Low appetite.

- Day 4: Mating cycle was triggered during morning sleep. Woke up at sunrise.  Headache all day long. Stayed in bed most of the day.

- Day 5: Milder headache and lethargic.  In bed in the afternoon with headache.  The headache seemed to increase as I was taking the four doses of L-Carnitine L-Tartrate during the day.  Right earache during the evening that subsided by bedtime.

- Day 6: Mild headache that subsided by lunchtime. Afternoon fatigue.  Altitude test to 4,024 feet.  No symptoms of altitude hypersensitivity.  Sore right knee joint when walking in the evening.

- Day 7: Woke up energized.  Fatigue onset as the day progressed that did not respond to caffeine.  Hungry in the evening and overeating.

- Day 8: Woke up at sunrise.  Fatigued and exhibiting confusion.  Altitude test to 6,632 feet.  No symptoms of altitude hypersensitivity.  Ears popping and skull pains.

- Day 9: Feeling fine.

The dose was raised to what the manufacturer recommended, as I was concerned that I may not be taking enough of it to fully treat the altitude hypersensitivity.  Based on the above symptoms, there was a profound response to the increased dosing which I took as an indication that a deficiency was being corrected in the body.

I removed the Amberen to see if the L-Carnitine L-Tartrate could treat altitude hypersensitivity on its own.

Research into L-Carnitine L-Tartrate indicated that 3,000 mg is considered the safe level of maximum dosing in adults. Given the profound reactions I was having to it, I decided to do a couple of weeks at 3 doses daily of 1,000 mg. The following reactions were seen at the maximum dosing level:

- Day 1: Insomnia until 1 am.

- Day 2: Woke up fatigued. Coffee cleared it. Had good energy levels and concentration.

- Day 3: Had good energy levels and concentration.

- Day 4: Fatigued PM.

- Day 5: Feeling fine. Altitude test to 2,000 feet. No symptoms of altitude hypersensitivity.

- Day 6: Feeling fine.

- Day 7 to 10: Started to develop mild headaches.

- Day 11: Altitude test to 4,024 feet. Mild headache that progressed into severe headache at altitude. Showing increasing confusion during the drive. Started Amberen to treat the headache and confusion. Both subsided during sleep.

- Day 12: At 140 feet above sea level. Fatigued in the morning that responded to caffeine.

- Day 13: Altitude test to 6,632 feet. Feeling normal. Mild headache during altitude exposure. Cleared up at sea level in Kona. No further issues on the drive home at 1,000 to 2,000 feet. Slept at 600 feet.

- Day 14: Mild skull pains.

- Day 15: Back to normal.

Removing Amberen did cause altitude hypersensitivity to return.  It was also accompanied by headaches.  Taking the Amberen cleared up both conditions.  It appears the altitude exposure is needed for nutritional absorption throughout the body, including the brain.

There appears to be two supplements needed to keep altitude hypersensitivity treated once it has been cleared and that is:

- L-Carnitine L-Tartrate at 500 mg to 3,000 mg daily.
  - Bulk Supplements.
- Amberen.
  - Biogix, Inc.

L-Carnitine and Amberen were working together to clear up the altitude hypersensitivity.  There is an interaction taking place between them and one does not work without the other.

I have remained free of most food intolerance using only L-Carnitine L-Tartrate.  Mental and physical health were good.  Energy levels were good.

Regarding the rest of the supplements, it seems they reduce the altitude hypersensitivity, but they do not fully clear it up like the L-Carnitine and Amberen do.  Given the rest of the supplements improve sex, it appears they are treating deficiencies within the body.

The key suspected ingredients that treat altitude hypersensitivity were L-Carnitine and glycine.  Research revealed a supplement that had both of these in it called "Glycine Propionyl-L-Carnitine (GPLC)".  I purchased the following GPLC products:

- Carlyle GPLC Supplement 1250mg.
  - Propionyl-L-Carnitine 824 mg.
  - Glycine 282 mg.
  - CoQ10 60 mg.

- VitaMonk GlycoTrax.
  - Glycine Propionyl-L-Carnitine 1,000 mg.


L-Carnitine and Amberen were removed and were replaced by GPLC.  My body remained free of altitude hypersensitivity during altitude tests.  I took GPLC for three months and did not see altitude hypersensitivity return during that time.

There was a notable difference in the GPLC supplements.  Carlyle GPLC was unstable and would degrade after opening the supplement container.  When I would put it in my pill box, by the end of a week the Carlyle GPLC capsules would be degrading.  After a couple of months in the pill bottle, they were unusable.  I threw the last few capsules I had away.  No such issues were observed with VitaMonk GlycoTrax.  The Carlyle GPLC appeared to be the better GPLC supplement for treating altitude hypersensitivity and this reflected its higher level of GPLC.

These are my conclusions about treating my altitude hypersensitivity:

- Low protein organic diet.

- Base nutritional supplements are L-Carnitine and glycine.

- Optimized nutrition through appropriate supplementation and diet.


There is currently no known cure for altitude hypersensitivity, it appears to be a lifelong treatment.  It may be arising in the general population from flying, mountain activities, living at altitude, lung damage, man-made environmental changes, climate change and new bacteria and viruses.

*"I was surprised at how simple the treatment for Altitude Hypersensitivity was."*

**Steven Magee**

## **Altitude Sickness**

There are five different ranges of altitudes that altitude sickness falls into:

1.  Sea Level:
    - A damaged body in a state of altitude sickness at sea level.
    - Acclimatization never occurs.

2.  Altitude Hypersensitivity:
    - Above sea level to 4,900 feet.
    - Acclimatization only occurs below the "Altitude Hypersensitivity Threshold" where symptoms are not observed.

3.  High Altitude:
    - 4,900 to 11,500 feet.

4.  Very High Altitude:
    - 11,500 to 18,000 ft.

5.  Extreme Altitude:
    - Above 18,000 ft.

Hypoxia ties altitude sickness, COVID-19 and long COVID together.  The symptoms to look out for are:

- Headache.

- Confusion.

- Fatigue.

- Stomach illness.

- Dizziness.

- Sleep disturbance.

- Central sleep apnea.

- Exertion may aggravate the symptoms.


If you are experiencing any of the above symptoms, you may need to move to a rural sea level area to recover.  If you are unable to move, then altitude sickness supplements and/or treatments may be able to improve your health.  More information can be found in the book "Toxic Altitude" by Steven Magee.


*"After my flu-like illness, I was telling the doctors my progressing sickness felt like Altitude Sickness!"*

**Steven Magee**

## **Pandemic Supplements 1**

This was the first supplementation system I developed for treating my long COVID symptoms:

Steven Magee takes daily:

- Daily multivitamin.
  - Kirkland Signature.
- Calcium citrate, magnesium and zinc.
  - Kirkland Signature.
- Wild alaskan salmon oil 1,000 mg.
  - Pure Alaska Omega.
- Betaine HCl, pepsin and genetian bitters.
  - Doctor's best.
- Vitamin B12 5,000 mcg.
  - Kirkland Signature.
- Vitamin C 1,000 mg.
  - Kirkland Signature.
- Vitamin D 10,000 IU.
  - Carlyle.
- Alpha Lipoic Acid 300 mg.
  - Puritan's Pride.
- Folic acid 400 mcg.
  - Sundown.
- Iron 65 mg.
  - Nature Made.

- Creatine Monohydrate 3 g.
  - Now Sports.
- Amino acid drink 10 g.
  - Essential amino energy by Optimum Nutrition.
- L-Citrulline 6 g.
  - Bulk Supplements.
- L-Lysine-HCL 1.5 g.
  - Bulk Supplements.
- Acetyl-L-Carnitine HCI 750 mg.
  - Jacked Factory.
- L-Arginine 500 mg.
  - Jacked Factory.
- Amberen.
  - Biogix, Inc.
- Testosterone Support one capsule.
  - Weider Prime.
- Extreme Test one capsule.
  - Influx Inspire.
- Breakfast is a pot of coffee (12 cups - 60 ounces) slowly consumed between sunrise and noon.
  - Kirkland Signature whole bean french roast coffee.
  - Kirkland Signature organic coffee creamer french vanilla flavored.

The iron tablet can be replaced with an iron fish, which may be more effective in the long term. "Kirkland" branded products are obtained at Costco.

The supplements are taken at breakfast, around 7 am. Missing a dose of the supplements generally causes sleepiness and fatigue to occur by 3 pm onward. This can be offset by taking the missed supplements. If the missed supplements are not taken until the next morning, then a progressive feeling of sickness will occur during the night. Taking the supplements the next morning clears the sickness.

Regarding food intake, I only drink liquids in the morning until noon. Breakfast is coffee and creamer. Lunch and dinner are solids and they are eaten between noon and 6pm. Food and drink intake is as follows:

- Sunrise: Wake up and spend 30 minutes outdoors.

- Morning: Take supplements with coffee and creamer.

- Noon: Start eating solids for lunch.

- 5pm: Solids dinner.

- 6pm: Start fasting, drink water only if needed.

- Sunset: Watch sunset for light absorption into the body to prepare it for sleep.

- Once the onset of tiredness takes place, go to bed with the curtains open for starlight, planet and moonlight exposures during sleep. The head of the bed needs to be under the window so that nighttime light can shine onto the face.

- Food fasting starts at 6pm and goes through to sunrise the next day.

- Liquids fast is typically 12 hours long.

- Liquids are only consumed for approximately 12 hours per day.

- Solids fast is typically 18 hours long.

- Solids are only eaten for 6 hours per day.

The supplements need to be taken in conjunction with daily outdoor exercise.  That exercise should be a mix of cardio and muscle building exercise that is done for at least an hour.  Vigorous swimming, lifting weights and/or cycling hills are effective. Regular sex is an excellent cardio exercise.

Long term testing over several months revealed the side effects of this supplement plan:

- Nerve damage at 9,200 feet occurred after an altitude test. (May not be related to the supplements.)

- Sore knees.

- Cramping in the right foot and right hand.

*"Nutritional supplements had far more beneficial effects than any of the prescription drugs."*

**Steven Magee**

## **Minimum Supplements**

One of the things I like to do is find out what are the minimum amount of supplements I need to take to maintain improved health.  As such, I removed some of supplements I thought were non-essential at the time to see if I would continue in good health.  The following were removed in August 2022:

- Daily multivitamin.
  - Kirkland Signature.

- Wild alaskan salmon oil 1,000 mg.
  - Pure Alaska Omega.

- Betaine HCI, pepsin and genetian bitters.
  - Doctor's best.

- Creatine Monohydrate 3 g.
  - Now Sports.

- Acetyl-L-Carnitine HCI 750 mg.
  - Jacked Factory.

- L-Arginine 500 mg.
  - Jacked Factory.

I did see an adverse reaction to removing Creatine Monohydrate.  It caused severe sensitivity in my teeth, it was so severe that I could only eat liquid foods after five days of not taking it.  The sensitive teeth subsided after two weeks.  Stopping Acetyl-L-Carnitine HCI did bring on sensitive teeth for a couple of days.

The reduced supplements did have a negative effect on sexual functioning and reintroducing the full range of supplements fixed it.  I had better sex and sexual stamina on the full range of supplements.

*"It is important to experiment with supplements to verify you actually need to take them.  Taking a non-essential supplement is just wasting your money."*

**Steven Magee**

## **Pandemic Supplements 2**

This supplement plan was developed to eliminate the knee pains that the first one was causing.  It was suspected the knee pains were coming from supplement toxicity, so known toxic supplements were removed.  Some supplements that were thought not to be needed anymore were also removed.  The removed supplements did clear up the knee pains.

Steven Magee takes daily:

- Daily multivitamin.
    - Kirkland Signature.
- Calcium citrate, magnesium and zinc.
    - Kirkland Signature.
- Wild alaskan salmon oil 1,000 mg.
    - Pure Alaska Omega.
- Vitamin C 1,000 mg.
    - Kirkland Signature.
- Amino acid drink 10 g.
    - Essential amino energy by Optimum Nutrition.
- L-Citrulline 6 g.
    - Bulk Supplements.
- L-Lysine-HCL 1.5 g.
    - Bulk Supplements.
- Acetyl-L-Carnitine HCI 750 mg.
    - Jacked Factory.
- L-Arginine 500 mg.

- ○ Jacked Factory.
- Amberen.
  - ○ Biogix, Inc.
- Testosterone Support one capsule.
  - ○ Weider Prime.
- Extreme Test one capsule.
  - ○ Influx Inspire.
- Breakfast is a pot of coffee (12 cups - 60 ounces) slowly consumed between sunrise and noon.
  - ○ Kirkland Signature whole bean french roast coffee.
  - ○ Kirkland Signature organic coffee creamer french vanilla flavored.
- Kidney Cleanse as needed.
  - ○ Dr. Bo.

Sexual performance was excellent with long lasting sex sessions. It was further improved by doubling the dose of the testosterone boosting supplements.

A kidney cleanse was performed during this supplement protocol due to recognizing that the kidneys were involved in the amino acid deficiencies I have.

*"It is important to know which supplements you are taking are associated with toxicity to the human."*

**Steven Magee**

## **Pandemic Supplements 3**

This set of supplements was for improved nail and skin growth.  I was still having fungal toenail growth and I was suspicious the fungal infection was systemic.  I had a history of skin tags on my body after my flu-like illness that brought on long COVID symptoms.  Research indicated the most effective treatment for fungal nails was an oral anti-fungal medication.  This set of supplements was developed to attempt to counteract a systemic fungal infection.

The Amberen and L-Carnitine were removed, as I wanted to see if they could be replaced by GPLC to treat altitude hypersensitivity.  Testing went well with GPLC and it does effectively treat altitude hypersensitivity.

The amino acid powders were removed to make it easier to travel.  Traveling through airports with white powdered amino acids may flag you up to TSA as a suspected drugs dealer.  I have had this experience in Kona airport in Hawaii and it is unpleasant! They tested all of the powders for drugs and it delayed me going through TSA!  It was all done in front of the passengers going through the TSA area, so the passengers know what is going on.  I got some strange looks from passengers once I was inside the airport gate area!

Two weeks after the amino acid powders were removed, the food sensitivities came back.  I was getting very sleepy after some large evening meals.  I introduced a 1,000 mg tablet of L-Arginine daily and within a few days, the food sensitivities were reduced but not completely gone.  Adding Citrulline to it brought on headaches but did not clear up the food sensitivities.  I happened to drink a can of "Monster Energy" with my morning supplements that I had got free with a purchase at a store.  This completely cleared the headaches up!

Why would "Monster Energy" clear up the headaches?  It has some extra supplements in it that were not in my regular daily supplements:

- Taurine.

- Panax Ginseng.

- L-Carnitine L-Tartrate.

- Guarana.

- Other ingredients.


There is something in this drink that interacted with my supplements to clear up the headaches.  It required just one 16 fluid ounces can to be taken with the morning supplements.  I suspect the "Monster Energy" was acting as a catalyst that increased or altered the pre-existing chemistry of my supplements.  It triggered a beneficial reaction that only required one dose.  Once the reaction had occurred, my existing supplements were sufficient at preventing headaches and they did not return.   The ingredients in "Monster Energy" has commonality with some of the supplements that were used in the pandemic supplement protocols described in this book.

Food intolerance was still present in the evening after eating a large evening meal, bringing on tiredness and sleepiness.  Mental functioning was beginning to decline and I was starting to feel weird brain functioning.  It seemed the travel supplements were not fully treating the nutritional deficiencies I had.

The home where I was staying had a canister of "Amino Energy" and decided to start taking the full recommended dose of six scoops daily.  I would take two scoops as soon as I woke up, another two scoops mid-morning and the final two scoops at lunchtime.  This cleared up the food intolerance and brain functioning issues after one week.

Adjusting to six scoops daily of "Amino Energy" did bring on the following conditions in the first week:

- Nerve pains.
- Dreams.

Once the adjustment took place, the symptoms subsided and I was feeling good again!  Lots of energy daily, no fatigue and good mental functioning.

The "Amino Energy" powder was replaced with amino acid tablets called "Amino Acid Complex 3000mg" by Horbaach. There was a mild headache reaction after several days that lasted for a day and cleared with sleep.  I did get a brief period where I could remember dreaming for a few days.  I remained free of symptoms and had developed a tablet based amino acid supplementation protocol that worked for me.

I stopped taking the multivitamin and replaced it with B-complex.  This was due to being on the multivitamin for almost a year and I wanted to take a break from it.

I decided to replace the calcium citrate, magnesium and zinc with just magnesium and to increase the dose.  This was due to seeing an increase in sleeping oxygen events.   I took the magnesium up to 250 mg from 80 mg daily.

The supplement system did not feel quite right, so a little research on it revealed it was very similar to what is being used to treat autistic children.  Zinc is a big feature of that treatment.  As such, I raised the zinc levels by adding a 50 mg zinc tablet daily. The reviews of the zinc supplement were showing 50 mg daily was well tolerated by most people.

Memory and confusion had slowly increased during developing this supplement protocol and had subsided once it had been fully developed.

The increased levels of the amino acids in the prior supplement protocols appear to improve sexual functioning. Adding in the zinc brought on morning erections and improved things.  Sexual functioning waned during development of this supplement protocol before normalizing once completed.

Steven Magee takes daily:

- Magnesium Citrate 250 mg.
  - Nature Made.
- Zinc 50 mg.
  - Nature's Bounty.
- Wild alaskan salmon oil 1,000 mg.
  - Pure Alaska Omega.
- Super B complex with vitamin C one tablet.
  - CVS Health.
- Vitamin C 2,000 mg.
  - Kirkland Signature.
- Vitamin E 180 mg.
  - Kirkland Signature.
  - For external use.  Paint one capsule onto affected fungal nails and skin daily after showering.
- Vitamin E 1,440 mg.
  - Kirkland Signature.
- Biotin 10,000 mcg.
  - Bronson.
- GPLC two capsules.
  - Carlyle.
- L-Arginine & L-Citrulline one tablet.
  - Amazing Nutrition.
- Amino Acid Complex three tablets.
  - Horbaach.
- Testosterone Support one capsule.

- ○ Weider Prime.
- Extreme Test one capsule.
  - ○ Influx Inspire.
- Organic greek yogurt plain one tablespoon with each meal.
  - ○ Kirkland.
- Breakfast is a pot of coffee (12 cups - 60 ounces) slowly consumed between sunrise and noon.
  - ○ Kirkland Signature whole bean french roast coffee.
  - ○ Full cream milk.
- "Monster Energy" 16 fluid ounces if needed.
  - ○ Monster Energy Company.

Sore shoulders and neck were observed in the first few weeks of taking this supplement combination and it slowly subsided.  It was suspected to be the adjustment to the high dose of vitamin E.  The area of my upper back and neck soreness were consistent with the area associated with Kyphosis.  Kyphosis is an abnormally excessive convex curvature of the spine as it occurs in the thoracic and sacral regions.

Stools were looser on this supplement protocol and it was thought to be the anti-fungal properties of vitamin E that were affecting the contents of the digestive tract.  Daily morning defecations were easy and pleasant.

Improved nail and hair growth was observed during the time I have been taking this supplement protocol.  At three months into high dosing of vitamin E I was not noticing any side effects or toxicity associated with it.  Vitamin E toxicity showed up in me during the fourth month of high daily dosing.  It was a sensation of not feeling well with brain fog.  Pulse oximeter testing showed that my heart rate was elevated by about 30 beats per minute (BPM) more than normal.  Stopping the vitamin E cleared the toxicity and restored the natural heart rate.  Withdrawal symptoms were mild and included some insomnia, dizziness and aches and pains in the following weeks.

I was free of food intolerance symptoms and could eat a normal diet. I was not avoiding any food types. I could eat a huge pepperoni pizza from Costco without any issues.

This supplement system produced the highest energy levels. I was very alert and capable on it. A lot of jobs were getting done on my home!

After I wrapped up research on pandemic supplements 3, my supply of GPLC ran out. I noticed glycine was contained within the amino acid complex tablets and all I had to do was add in the L-Carnitine to replace the GPLC. I had L-Carnitine L-Tartrate from previous testing and I replaced the GPLC with it at a single 2 g daily dose. My body remained free of Altitude Hypersensitivity.

**"Traveling through airports with white powders may get you flagged by TSA as a potential drugs dealer!"**

**Steven Magee**

## **Supplement Overdose Symptoms**

During developing pandemic supplements I did experience two distinct symptoms of supplement overdosing:

- Changed taste – coffee did not taste right, regardless of brand.

- Aching joints.

It is important when taking supplements to research the side effects of them to know when you may be displaying them. Changing my pandemic supplement protocol from 1 to 2 did eliminate the sore joints. My taste remained changed and I expect that will not rectify itself until I reduce my supplements to a maintenance dose of just what is essential for me.

The changed taste had coincided with a virus that I had while traveling around the USA in October and November 2022. The virus did not test positive for COVID-19, although the symptoms were similar. I had a couple of days of mild flu-like symptoms with lung pains during sleeping. It cleared up and the only symptom I was left with was all types of coffee tasting bland. It all tasted the same to me regardless of brand or roast.

*"When taking nutritional supplements, it is important to know which ones have toxicity associated with them."*

**Steven Magee**

## **Medical Tests**

You should be aware that nutritional supplementing can affect the results of numerous medical tests.  It can hide medical conditions from detection.  Some of the test results known to be affected by nutritional supplements are:

- Thyroid hormone.

- Vitamin D.

- Calcium.

- Prostate specific-antigen (PSA).

- Hepatitis B.

- Hepatitis C.

- COVID-19.

- Heart attack.

- Bone density scans.

- Stool.

- Cardiac diseases.

- Endocrine disorders.

- Cancers.

- Anemias.

- Kidney disease.

- Infectious diseases.

The higher the doses of nutritional supplements are, the more likely they are to interfere with medical tests.  Known supplements that cause medical test problems are:

- Riboflavin (B2).

- Biotin (B7).

- Niacin.

- Vitamin B12.

- Vitamin C.

- Vitamin E.

- Calcium.

- Iron.

- L-tryptophan.

- St. John's wort.

- 5-HTP.

Other things that are known to affect medical test results are:

- Some foods.

- Some drinks.

- Intense physical activity.

- Sunburn.

- Colds

- Infections.

- Having sex.

- Some medications or drugs.

- Lack of sleep.

- Dehydration.

You should discuss your nutritional supplement intake with your doctor prior to ordering medical tests. You should query abnormal test results that may have been adversely affected by nutritional supplements. Both "false-positive" and "false-negative" test results are known to occur.

**"*Nutritional supplements may give you false or inaccurate results on medical laboratory tests.*"**

**Steven Magee**

## **Supplement Toxicity**

The following supplements are well known to have the ability to cause toxicity in the human:

- An excess of vitamin B6.

- Fat soluble vitamins A, D, E, and K.

- Iron tablets.

When taking supplements and noticing the onset of unusual health issues, it is wise to review the toxicity of the supplements you are taking.

*"Supplement toxicity in me was causing sore knees.  I removed the suspected supplements and the sore knees disappeared!"*

**Steven Magee**

## Summary

So what have I learned since I have been researching supplements?  The human body accumulates damage as it ages from environmental exposures, injuries and infections.  Altitude sickness and coronavirus infections are very similar and can cause comparable damage throughout the body from hypoxia.  It can make a person sensitized to just a small change in altitude or air pressure.  Nutritional supplements can offset some of this damage by correcting malnutrition issues in the body and detoxifying toxins the damaged body is producing.

It is no secret the medical profession struggles with long COVID patients.  They appear to stay sickly under their care and throwing prescription drugs and medical devices at their unusual health conditions can make them sicker!  Many of my long COVID symptoms were misdiagnosed during years of visits to numerous doctors.  I was never referred to a nutritionist, despite having serious food intolerance for years.

The mental health profession were very disappointing.  I was surprised at how bad they were!  They will diagnose you with a range of mental health conditions and start prescribing you potent brain drugs.  When you tell them the brain drugs are making you sicker, they tell you to take more!  The treatment was so bad from them that I had to stop using them to protect my own health and safety!

Mental illness is a common diagnosis that doctors fall back onto when they do not understand what is wrong with the patient. You need to be very careful about interacting with doctors with this diagnosis.  If you start talking about poisoning with them, they may say it is your mental illness making you paranoid and you may get locked up in the mental health hospital!  Be very careful about your interactions with doctors once you have a mental illness diagnosis!  They have the power to institutionalize you.

I was attending an army of doctors from 2015 to 2021 with long COVID symptoms.  Many were at the university research hospital.  They could not accurately diagnose me.  What was I telling them?  The sickness I have feels like altitude sickness!  I have looked up my symptoms and it matches poisoning!  They could not diagnose altitude hypersensitivity and ammonia poisoning.  Nothing showed up on their many medical tests to indicate these conditions were present.  This is how my treatment went:

- Lung damage and asthma was treated with numerous inhalers.  The actual treatment was to move to a rural sea level area.

- Sleep apnea and bruxism were treated with an anti-back device, stimulants, CPAP and BiPAP machines.  The CPAP and BiPAP machines had been given to me with the pressure setting too high and were actually making me sicker!  The actual treatment was to move to sea level, sleep on my front and take magnesium.

- Mental illness was treated with potent brain drugs.  The actual treatment was to identify the altitude hypersensitivity and ammonia poisoning, take amino acids and move to sea level.

- Fatigue was treated with stimulants.  The actual treatment was to identify nutritional deficiencies, food intolerance and disrupted circadian rhythms, and take amino acids, move to sea level and live in a tent outside for several months.

- Heart arrhythmia was being treated with numerous prescription medications.  The actual treatment was nutritional support for the heart and move to sea level.

- Gastrointestinal problems were treated with a colonoscopy and removal of a polyp.  They got part of the treatment right.  The full treatment was live culture support from yogurt, nutritional support, daily exercise, a cooler environment and move to sea level.

- Fungal toenails were treated by removing the toenails and painting an anti-fungal onto the new nails which did not work. The correct treatment appears to be an oral anti-fungal for several months, painting an anti-fungal onto the toenails, treating the ammonia poisoning and move to sea level.

- Food intolerance was never treated. The correct treatment was to adopt a comprehensive nutritional support system that included amino acids, a low protein diet and move to sea level.

- Altitude sickness was never treated. The correct treatment was to move to sea level and take L-Carnitine and glycine.

- Poisoning was never treated. The correct treatment was arginine, citrulline and lysine nutritional supplementation, detoxify from heavy metals poisoning and move to sea level.

My treatment from the doctors ranged from almost nothing through to lots of prescription drugs. The treatment varied between each doctor. Some were watching how my health was degrading and monitoring it, while others were trying to use prescription drugs to fix it. I had one doctor that was trying to tell me it was "All in my mind!". I left that doctor after hearing that.

Be aware the modern medical profession has no real incentive to fix you. Financially, the doctor is in a much better position if you stay sick, because you will be a regular at the office and will be producing a nice income for the doctor!

There are no doubts that the modern medical system is under the influence of pharmaceutical companies. Many of their expensive drugs work no better than nutritional supplements! But the prescriptions may come with nasty side effects. Some of my prescription medications were $500 per month for each medicine!

By the time I was done with the medical profession in 2021, I had been under the care of numerous primary care doctors, numerous specialist doctors and I had been attending the four main hospitals in Tucson including the university research hospital.

At the age of fifty-three I will never be cured of permanent biological damage. I was fortunate I had some lucky breaks that improved my mental functioning to the point I could correctly self diagnose my symptoms. One of these was my ex-girlfriend switching out my diet to a gluten free one. Had this not happened, I would still be misdiagnosed!

I call my disease "Magee's Disease", as I have not been able to find a medical condition in the published medical literature that covers the full range of health issues I had. As such, I believe Magee's disease is a new and previously undocumented health condition in the general population. This explains why all of the numerous doctors I saw were unable to make a diagnosis of Magee's disease and prescribe the correct treatment.

My recovery has been so successful that I have not been to a doctors office since I left Arizona in July 2021. I have medical insurance in Hawaii and I have never needed to use it in almost two years. I do not have a primary care doctor. At the peak of the sickness in Tucson, I was averaging a doctors visit every few weeks! I was under the care of a wide range of specialist doctors at the time.

My other books provide further information on health and you may want to consider reading them:

- Pandemic Supplements.

- Magee's Disease.

- Curing Electromagnetic Hypersensitivity.

- Toxic Altitude.

- Toxic Electricity.

- Toxic Health.

- Toxic Light.

- Solar Radiation, Global Warming, and Human Disease.

I hope you enjoyed this book and I wish you the very best of health.

153

*"I was surprised the USA medical profession could not diagnose low blood oxygen levels, sensitivity to abnormal air, food intolerance, malnutrition, a urea cycle disorder, altitude hypersensitivity, loss of circadian rhythm and loss of moonlight synchronization."*

**Steven Magee**

# References

**Books:**

- Brain Longevity by Dharma Singh Khalsa.

- Brain Maker: The Power of Gut Microbes to Heal and Protect Your Brain - for Life by David Perlmutter with Kristin Loberg.

- HEAVY METALS DETOX: The fast-track to a healthier version of YOU! by James Lilley.

- No Grain, No Pain: A 30-Day Diet for Eliminating the Root Cause of Chronic Pain by Peter Osborne.

- Prescription For Nutritional Healing by James F. Balch, MD & Phyllis A Balch, CNC.

- The Complete Low-FODMAP Diet: A Revolutionary Plan for Managing IBS and Other Digestive Disorders by Sue Shepherd.

- The Plant Paradox - The Hidden Dangers in "Healthy" Foods That Cause Disease and Weight Gain by Dr. Steven R Gundry MD.

- Wheat Belly by William Davis.

**Internet:**

- Dietary supplement:
  - https://en.wikipedia.org/wiki/Dietary_supplement

- Linus Pauling Institute's Micronutrient Information Center:
  - https://lpi.oregonstate.edu/mic/

- NIH Dietary Supplement Fact Sheets:

- - https://ods.od.nih.gov/factsheets/list-all/
- Mayo Clinic nutrition and healthy eating:
  - https://www.mayoclinic.org/healthy-lifestyle/nutrition-and-healthy-eating/basics/nutrition-basics/hlv-20049477

- The Nutrition Source at Harvard College:
  - https://www.hsph.harvard.edu/nutritionsource/

- WebMD Vitamins & Supplements:
  - https://www.webmd.com/vitamins/index


*"I found my correct diagnosis in books and on the internet."*

**Steven Magee**

## **Most At Risk Of Hypoxia**

The most at risk of hypoxia illnesses and diseases are:

- Space.
  - Astronauts.
  - Tourists.
- Aviation workers.
  - Pilots.
  - Airline cabin crew.
  - Frequent fliers.
- High altitude astronomy workers.
- Winter sports.
  - Skiers.
  - Snowboarders.
- Mountain hikers.
- High altitude hikers.
- Mountain workers.
  - Lodges.
  - Resorts.
  - Some national parks.
- Forest workers.
- People that live in altitude cities.
- Drivers and truckers.
- Radio and television transmitter workers.
- Cell phone tower workers.

- People with pre-existing health conditions.

- People with sea level adapted genetics.

- People with a hole in the heart (ASD).

- People that have breathed industrial gasses.

- People that have breathed medical gasses.

- People that live inside poorly ventilated homes with gas appliances.

- People that have been exposed to hypoxic environments.

- People that have had a coronavirus infection.

- People with Long COVID.

*"Truckers that drive all over the USA are often in hypoxic environments!"*

**Steven Magee**

## Acknowledgments

This book was influenced by:

- Those that are developing the important science of environmental health and bringing it to the masses.

- My family for providing support during my prolonged and mysterious illness.

*"Mysterious disabling illnesses will make you dependent on people."*

**Steven Magee**

## **About The Author**

About Steven Magee CEng MIET BEng Hons, member of Environmental Radiation LLC:

Steven was born in the United Kingdom (UK) and started his career at one of the largest university research and teaching hospitals in Europe. Working in the electrical engineering group, he obtained a Bachelors with Honors in Electrical and Electronic Engineering. Human health was a strong draw and he moved into the biomedical team, serving the regions hospitals. During this time he developed a fascination for human illness and disease and the causes of it, many of which were not understood.

He joined the Isaac Newton Group of Telescopes in 1999 and went to live in La Palma. La Palma is part of the Canary Islands, governed by Spain. During this time he worked with the leading European astronomers and developed his astronomical and optics skills. He became fluent in Spanish and their culture.

In 2001 he became a Chartered Electrical Engineer and joined the W. M. Keck Observatory in Hawaii. This was the world's leading astronomical facility and home to the world's two largest segmented mirror telescopes. Steven developed segmented optics and interferometry skills while working alongside world leading astronomers. He was the assistant to Nobel Prize winners including the fourth woman to win the prize in physics, Andrea Ghez. During this time Steven constructed his own off-grid solar powered home in the last of the traditional Hawaiian fishing villages in Miloli'i, Hawaii. He learned Hawaiian Pidgin English and the Hawaiian culture during his time there.

In 2006, Steven became the Director of the MDM Observatory in Sells, Arizona, USA. Working for Columbia University and later, Dartmouth College, he developed the facility to modern standards. He learned an appreciation of the Native Americans and their culture from the Tohono O'odham Nation.

In 2008, Steven joined the solar power revolution that was sweeping the USA and commissioned the largest CIGS thin film solar photovoltaic installation in the world.

A year later he became the Florida Power and Light (FPL) Manager of the DeSoto Next Generation Solar Energy Center, which was the largest solar photovoltaic utility power generation plant ever built in the USA. The system rated power was quoted as 25,000,000 watts AC with over 90,500 solar modules that were mounted to 158 single-axis tracker systems in three hundred acres of land and it was opened by President Obama.

He went on to develop the solar photovoltaic team for a large international company.

In 2010 he started to research radiation and publish the leading books on the subject.

He became a USA citizen in 2017 and continues to be interested in global radiation health effects and how it impacts over seven billion people on planet Earth.

*"I had a very interesting career that sent me into ill health and onto disability."*

**Steven Magee**

## **Author Contact**

This is the Environmental Radiation LLC website:

- www.environmentalradiation.com

You can follow the Twitter feed at:

- Steven Magee @EnvironmentEMR

- https://twitter.com/EnvironmentEMR

The Facebook page is:

- https://www.facebook.com/EnvironmentEMR

You may find my other books useful:

Altitude Sickness

- **Magee's Disease:** Magee's Disease, Summit Brain, Altitude Sickness, COVID-19 and Long COVID are all related. This book delves into the silent world of hypoxia and what it can do to people. The failings of the modern medical profession are examined and solutions to the hypoxic Magee's Disease are explored.

- **Summit Brain:** Summit Brain is a term used to describe the health issues that appear in people that commute to very high altitude. This book explores the biological reasons that cause Summit Brain to occur. Recovery from Summit Brain can be achieved and solutions are explored for underlying conditions that doctors may have missed.

<u>Architecture</u>

- **Solar Reflections for Architects, Engineers, and Human Health**: This book is a comprehensive collection of images, diagrams, and notes that document the effects of sunlight in architecture. This is essential information for architects, engineers, and the medical profession. The discovery of the "Multiple-Sun" effect in architecture is detailed and this book is illustrated in color.

<u>Circadian Rhythms & Sleep Disorders</u>

- **Night Shift Recovery:** Unusual work shifts may lead to the development of Shift Work Disorder. Shift work is well known for its ability to degrade human health. Recovery can be achieved and solutions are explored for underlying conditions that doctors may have missed.

<u>Climate Change</u>

- **Solar Radiation, Global Warming, and Human Disease**: This book examines the modern development of the Earth and the potential impacts on global warming and human disease. The destruction of the forests for modern agricultural use appears to have effects that are not fully understood and these are explored. Radiation deficiency and radiation overloading are investigated to see if they are factors in many illnesses and diseases.

## Human Health

- **Hypoxia, Mental Illness & Chronic Fatigue**: This book examines the many aspects of hypoxia that may lead to the development of mental illness and chronic fatigue. Modern society is filled with hypoxia experiences that are well known for their ability to affect brain functioning and energy levels. Solutions are explored for underlying conditions that doctors may have missed.

- **Solar Radiation – A Cause of Illness and Cancer?** Illness and cancers have become part of our modern culture. It has been discovered that extremely high levels of man-made solar radiation exist in modern society. Could this be the one of the causes of illness and cancers? This book examines the increase in solar radiation and applies it to human health.

## Nutrition

- **COVID Supplements:** Steven Magee became disabled by a mystery flu-like sickness he caught from an international university professor. During the COVID-19 pandemic, he realized his mysterious range of symptoms matched a new sickness called Long COVID. This book explores the science behind the nutritional supplements he used to recover his mental and physical health.

- **Pandemic Supplements:** Steven Magee became disabled by a mystery flu-like sickness he caught from an international university professor. During the COVID-19 pandemic, he realized his mysterious range of symptoms matched a new sickness called Long COVID. This book explores the nutritional supplements he used to recover his mental and physical health.

<u>Toxicity</u>

- **Toxic Altitude:**  Toxic Altitude explores the biological reasons that cause Altitude Sickness to occur in sea level adapted humans.  Recovery from the long term effects of Altitude Sickness can be achieved and solutions are explored for underlying conditions that doctors may have missed.

- **Toxic Electricity:**  Random aches and pains?  Fatigue?  Insomnia?  Facial pains?  Irregular heartbeats?  Sick kids?  Relationship problems?  Blotchy skin?  Anxiety? Toxic electricity takes a look at the electrical system and asks the question:  Is this one of the most toxic endeavors that humanity has ever engaged in?

- **Toxic Health:**  Toxic Health takes a look at the pollution that may be in your local environment and relates it to the health problems that it can cause.  Pollution in the human environment is only just starting to be understood and something as innocent as light may be able to make you really ill!  There are many examples of commonplace items in your environment that may have the ability to affect your health.  In particular, we will investigate if modern city life is the most toxic thing of all to the modern human!

- **Toxic Light:**  Toxic Light takes a look at the light pollution that may be in your local environment and relates it to the health problems that it may cause. Light in the human environment is only just starting to be understood and something as innocent as your sunglasses may be able to make you ill! There are many examples of commonplace items in your environment that may have the ability to affect your health. Get ready for enlightenment about the most important human nutrient of light!

Forensics

- **Electrical Forensics:** Electrical Forensics examines the many aspects of electricity, electronics and wireless communications that may lead to unusual behaviors to occur in humans. Electromagnetic interference is well known for its ability to affect mental functioning and human health. Electrical Forensics demonstrates how to identify toxic electromagnetic environments that may be the root cause of accidents and crimes.

- **Health Forensics:** Health Forensics examines the many aspects of modern society that may lead to unusual behaviors to occur in humans. Modern society has adopted habits that are well known for their ability to affect mental functioning and human health. Health Forensics demonstrates how to identify toxic human environments that may be the root cause of accidents and crimes.

- **Light Forensics**: Light Forensics examines the many aspects of modern lighting that may lead to unusual behaviors to occur in humans. Modern society has adopted optical products that are well known for their ability to affect mental functioning and human health. Light Forensics demonstrates how to identify toxic light that may be the root cause of accidents and crimes.


Religion

- **Solar Radiation, the Book of Revelations, and the Era of Light – Part 1:** Welcome to the Era of Light! Light has long been known to be essential nourishment for the human body. We will explore the different types of light that are present on Earth and relate it to human health and nature. Light is discussed extensively in the Bible and we will see if we can associate our findings to it. Finally, we will investigate if the Industrial Revolution has created the ultimate toxin of poisonous sunlight!


Professional


- **Engineering Science and Education Journal Volume: 11, Issue: 4, Active Control Systems for Large Segmented Optical Mirrors:** A new generation of optical telescopes is on the drawing board. These will be true giants with primary mirrors having a diameter of up to 100 meters. The technology that will enable this revolution to take place was developed at the W. M. Keck Observatory in Hawaii, where the world's largest segmented mirrors are in daily use. This article looks at how the W. M. Keck Observatory proved the mirror technology that will be behind this new generation of telescopes.


Solar Photovoltaic


- **Complete Solar Photovoltaics for Residential, Commercial, and Utility Systems:** Steven Magee has combined his three top selling books on solar power systems into one edition. Complete Solar Photovoltaics will train you on solar photovoltaics and show you how to design grid connected solar photovoltaic power systems. Operations and maintenance is detailed to enable you to have a complete understanding of solar photovoltaics from start to finish.

- **Solar Photovoltaics for Consumers, Utilities, and Investors:** This book details solar photovoltaic systems for consumers, utilities and investors. This would encompass residential, commercial and utility systems that are connected to the utility grid. There is a discussion of the different technologies available for the consumer and their advantages and disadvantages. For the utilities, there is invaluable advice on planning and constructing large projects. For the investor, forward looking statements try to predict the future of solar photovoltaics.

- **Solar Photovoltaic Training for Residential, Commercial, and Utility Systems:** This book details solar photovoltaic training for those who are interested in this area and also for those who are already working in the field. This would encompass residential, commercial, and utility systems that are connected to the utility grid. It is a comprehensive overview of a rapidly growing world of solar photovoltaic power generation technology.

- **Solar Photovoltaic Design for Residential, Commercial, and Utility Systems:** This book details how to design reliable solar photovoltaic power generation systems from a residential system, progressing to a commercial system, and finishing at the largest utility power generation systems. By following the guidelines in this book and your local solar photovoltaic electrical codes, you will be able to design trouble free solar power systems that give many years of reliable operation. When designed well, solar photovoltaic power generation is an excellent source of electrical power that results in much lower electricity bills, the power company will even refund you for the excess energy generated by your system if it is large enough. Building a grid tied solar power system is a relatively easy task. Given the large amount of government and electrical utility financial incentives that are available, it is a great time to join in the solar power revolution that is taking place in the world today.

- **Solar Photovoltaic Operation and Maintenance for Residential, Commercial, and Utility Systems:** This book details how to operate and maintain residential, commercial, and utility solar photovoltaic systems that are connected to the utility grid. By following the guidelines in this book you will be able to operate and maintain solar power systems that should give many years of reliable operation. Invaluable trouble shooting advice will aid in returning your system to full operation in the event of a problem.

- **Solar Photovoltaic DC Calculations for Residential, Commercial, and Utility Systems:** This book details how to run calculations for the DC circuit of solar photovoltaic systems. This would encompass residential, commercial, and utility systems that are connected to the utility grid. It covers the range of conditions that solar photovoltaic modules are exposed to throughout the year and shows how to incorporate these into an effective DC circuit that is well designed and reliable.

- **Solar Photovoltaic Resource for Residential, Commercial, and Utility Systems:** This book is a resource of information that is used in the solar photovoltaic field. This would encompass residential, commercial, and utility systems that are connected to the utility grid. It is a comprehensive collection of notes, diagrams, pictures and charts for a rapidly growing world of solar photovoltaic power generation technology. This book is illustrated in color.

Solar Radiation

- **Solar Irradiance and Insolation for Power Systems:** This book is a resource of information that is used in the solar power generation field. This would encompass residential, commercial, and utility systems that are connected to the utility grid. It is a comprehensive collection of notes, diagrams, pictures, and charts for a rapidly growing world of solar photovoltaic power generation technology. This book is illustrated in color.

- **Solar Site Selection for Power Systems:** This book is a comprehensive collection of images, diagrams, and notes that document the effects of light and heat in the solar power generation field. This would encompass residential, commercial, and utility systems that are connected to the utility grid. This is essential information for a rapidly growing world of solar power generation technology. This book is illustrated in color.

You can search "Steven Magee Books" for the very latest publications.

www.youtube.com videos supporting the ideas in the books can be found by searching StevenMageeBooks:

- https://www.youtube.com/user/StevenMageeBooks

*"Writing books is by far the most interesting thing I have done in life."*

**Steven Magee**

## Book Reviews

**Complete Solar Photovoltaics for Residential, Commercial, and Utility Systems** rated 5 out of 5 stars.

Reviewed by Amanda Bassett on December 4, 2015 titled "Perfect read".

Perfect for solar farm studies. Takes the reader from basics who doesn't know a sausage about electricity to turning it into a business. We are considering doing just this in Arizona ourselves.

**Curing Electromagnetic Hypersensitivity** rated 5 out of 5 stars.

Reviewed by Ann on on January 31, 2015 titled "Don't miss the message here folks!".

This book says a lot abut the importance of not only avoiding radiation but the necessity of taking steps to replenish and rebalance the body's own electrical system in order to build resistance to the unavoidable radiation exposures that we live with in this world.  I have suffered with EHS and MCS and over the years I have gotten the most improvement by tracking my nutrient/mineral levels and supplementing accordingly. I am not surprised that the author has gotten his health back by "charging his battery, " so to speak. I have always believed that the most effective way to prevent or cure disease is to improve the "terrain" of the body. Thanks to the author for pointing this out and sharing the specifics!

**Electrical Forensics** rated 5 out of 5 stars.

Review by John Puccetti on October 27, 2013 titled "Dangers of electricity"

Steven has made many of the health problems of our century known in his book. But what will we do is this information? We live in a corporate dictatorship that masquerades as democracy.

**Health Forensics** rated 5 out of 5 stars.

Reviewed by honesT on July 26, 2014 titled "Incredible insights you would have never thought of :O".

Incredible insights, seriously Steve nails it again. If your just an average person looking for some insight about the whole EMF thing this is for you 100%.  If your a seasoned EMF pro looking for some new insights this book is worth it`s weight in gold and you will, I have no doubt in my mind take in new knowledge that will no doubt open doors.  You do not have to read this book from cover to cover, just pick any chapter read and be amazed what you learn.  So many areas are covered in this book, it`s really like a mini encyclopedia for EMF and how that`s affecting our surroundings that in turn affect our body, mind and emotions.  I really can`t say enough I mean just look at the price it`s practically free :]

**Solar Photovoltaic Training for Residential, Commercial and Utility Systems** rated 5 out of 5 stars.

Reviewed by Kyle William Loshure on November 13, 2016 titled "Solar power is #1"

Thank you for your work!

**Solar Radiation, Global Warming and Human Disease** rated 5 out of 5 stars.

Reviewed by Donato Cobarrubias on October 4, 2014 titled "Five Stars"

Great book and great info! I learned a lot!

**Toxic Electricity** rated 5 out of 5 stars.

Review by Sam Wieder on December 13, 2013 titled "A Most Illuminating, Educational, and Helpful Book"

Toxic Electricity provides a clear and comprehensive description of the many ways in which electrical fields impact human health and offers simple steps that anyone can take to live a more vibrant life in our electrically toxic world. The author does a masterful job of presenting some fairly complex concepts in a way that is easily understandable. Reading this book will give you a deeper understanding of how unseen radiation in your living and working environment may be impacting you. If you've been battling different health challenges or are chronically tired for no apparent reason, this book may very well open your eyes to some answers that will help you regain your health and your life.

**Toxic Light** rated 5 out of 5 stars.

Titled "Five Stars".

Reviewed by Amazon Customer on September 17, 2018

Great book, lots of information about light you never hear about anywhere.

*"When I saw the five star reviews appearing, I knew the research was progressing in the right direction."*

**Steven Magee**

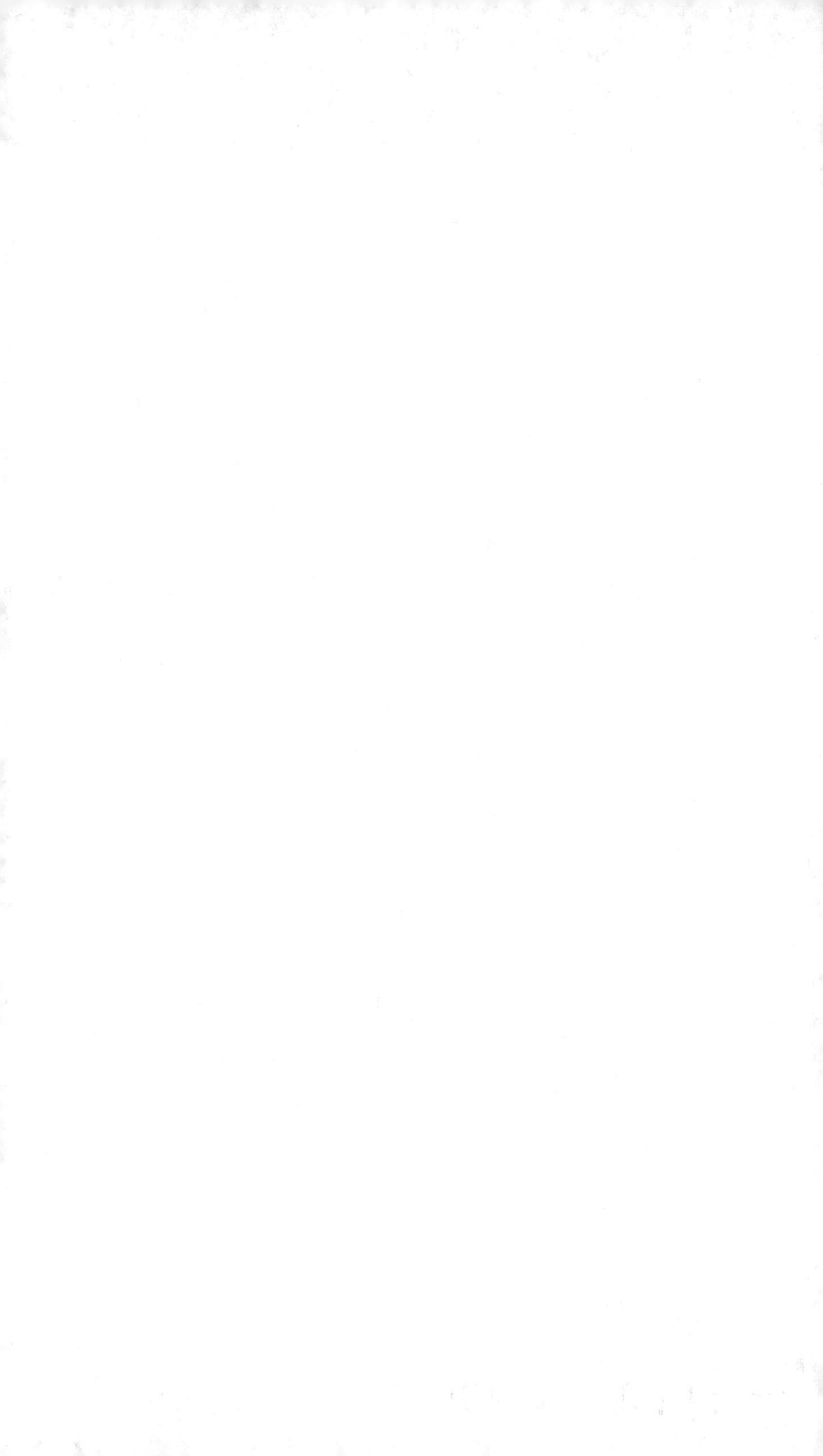